No More Joint Pain

Yale University Press Health & Wellness

A Yale University Press Health & Wellness book is an authoritative, accessible source of information on a health-related topic. It may provide guidance to help you lead a healthy life, examine your treatment options for a specific condition or disease, situate a healthcare issue in the context of your life as a whole, or address questions or concerns that linger after visits to your healthcare provider.

Joseph A. Abboud, M.D., and Soo Kim Abboud, M.D., *No More Joint Pain*

Thomas E. Brown, PH.D., *Attention Deficit Disorder: The Unfocused Mind in Children and Adults*

Marjorie Greenfield, M.D., *The Working Woman's Pregnancy Book*

Ruth H. Grobstein, M.D., PH.D., *The Breast Cancer Book: What You Need to Know to Make Informed Decisions*

James W. Hicks, M.D., *Fifty Signs of Mental Illness: A Guide to Understanding Mental Health*

Steven L. Maskin, M.D., *Reversing Dry Eye Syndrome: Practical Ways to Improve Your Comfort, Vision, and Appearance*

Mary Jane Minkin, M.D., and Carol V. Wright, PH.D., *A Woman's Guide to Menopause and Perimenopause*

Mary Jane Minkin, M.D., and Carol V. Wright, PH.D., *A Woman's Guide to Sexual Health*

Arthur W. Perry, M.D., F.A.C.S., *Straight Talk About Cosmetic Surgery*

Catherine M. Poole, with DuPont Guerry IV, M.D., *Melanoma: Prevention, Detection, and Treatment*, 2nd ed.

E. Fuller Torrey, M.D., *Surviving Prostate Cancer: What You Need to Know to Make Informed Decisions*

Barry L. Zaret, M.D., and Genell J. Subak-Sharpe, M.S., *Heart Care for Life: Developing the Program That Works Best for You*

No
More
Joint Pain

Joseph A. Abboud, M.D.,
and Soo Kim Abboud, M.D.

Yale University Press *New Haven and London*

The information and suggestions contained in this book are not intended to replace the services of your physician or caregiver. Because each person and each medical situation is unique, you should consult your own physician to get answers to your personal questions, to evaluate any symptoms you may have, or to receive suggestions for appropriate medications.

The authors have attempted to make this book as accurate and up to date as possible, but it may nevertheless contain errors, omissions, or material that is out of date at the time you read it. Neither the authors nor the publisher has any legal responsibility or liability for errors, omissions, out-of-date material, or the reader's application of the medical information or advice contained in this book.

Published with assistance from the foundation established in memory of Philip Hamilton McMillan of the Class of 1894, Yale College.

Designed by Gregg Chase
Set in by Ehrhardt by Tseng Information Systems, Inc.
Printed in the United States of America.
Library of Congress Cataloging-in-Publication Data
Abboud, Joseph A.
No more joint pain / Joseph A. Abboud and Soo Kim Abboud.
p. cm.—(Yale University Press health & wellness)
Includes bibliographical references and index.
ISBN 978-0-300-11175-0 (hardcover : alk. paper)
1. Joints—Diseases—Popular works. 2. Pain—Popular works. 3. Arthritis—Popular works.
I. Abboud, Soo Kim. II. Title.
RC932.A23 2008
616.7′2—dc22
2007039386
A catalogue record for this book is available from the British Library.
The paper in this book meets the guidelines for permanence and durability of the Committee on Production Guidelines for Book Longevity of the Council on Library Resources.
10 9 8 7 6 5 4 3 2 1

This book is dedicated to the memory of my father,
Albert Abboud, who taught me the importance of education,
perseverance, and intellectual curiosity

Contents

No More Joint Pain

The Many Causes of Joint Pain

THERE ARE ABOUT A hundred different forms of arthritis, an umbrella term for diseases with symptoms that include joint and musculoskeletal pain. And if you live long enough, you can pretty much count on developing symptoms of one of them—a touch of osteoarthritis, at the very least. In fact, more than 50 percent of people over age sixty-five have clinical signs of arthritis, meaning that an estimated seventy million Americans suffer from the disease. As the life expectancies for men and women continue to increase, Americans over the age of sixty-five will continue to be the most rapidly growing segment of the population. Consequently, according to even the most conservative estimates, the number of patients suffering from arthritis will nearly double by the year 2030 (a statistic that includes not only forms that emerge in the later years, but also those variations that affect young children, or adults in their prime). And osteoarthritis, the most prevalent form of arthritis, is the most common chronic disease affecting older individuals today.

Given this growing prevalence of osteoarthritis, it is not surprising that the health-care industry, which encompasses both traditional and unconventional modes of research and treatment, is rushing to develop and propose miracle cures—and that seniors who are confronted with arthritis can be all too ready to try them. After all, although Americans today look forward to living into and past their seventies and eighties, none imagine

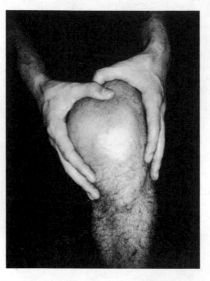

Almost everybody experiences joint pain at some point in their lifetime.

their golden years crippled with arthritis or envision their independence and quality of life hampered by other causes of joint pain. Our hope is that this book will help you become an educated health-care consumer — one who can easily distinguish among effective mainstream treatments, reasonable alternative treatments, and outright scams. In addition, while medical and surgical advances have given new hope to millions of joint pain and arthritis sufferers, this book will also stress the importance of arthritis prevention for readers who understand that early steps to avoid disease are always the best cure.

ANATOMY OF A JOINT

Human beings have more than one hundred joints connecting over two hundred bones, most of which are specifically designed to allow a broad range of motion. There are many different kinds of joints: ball-and-socket joints (think hips and shoulders), saddle joints (which connect thumb to hand), hinge joints (like those in your fingers and knees), or pivot joints (your wrists, for example).

In its simplest form, a joint is a connection between two or more bones and is made up of the ends of the bones; tough, rubbery cartilage that wraps around the ends of the two bones and that also functions as a shock absorber; a fluid-filled capsule that surrounds the bone ends and cartilage; and various ligaments and tendons that provide both stability

Arthritis Facts

• According to the Centers for Disease Control and Prevention, one in three adults in the United States suffers from arthritis or chronic joint pain.

• Almost twice as many women as men suffer from arthritis.

• Arthritis accounts for nearly forty million doctor visits and more than half a million hospitalizations.

• Osteoarthritis is the most common form of arthritis, afflicting more than twenty million Americans.

• Rheumatoid arthritis and gout are the second and third most common causes of arthritis. While rheumatoid arthritis strikes mostly women, gout tends to afflict men.

• Gout is twice as likely to strike African-American men as Caucasian men. This may be because more African-American men suffer from hypertension and take medication to lower their blood pressure. Some of these antihypertensive drugs can increase production of uric acid—the substance that crystallizes and then deposits in gouty joints.

• An astonishing 285,000 children under age seventeen have arthritis, including 50,000 who have juvenile rheumatoid arthritis.

and movement. Inside the joint capsule a special lining—the synovial membrane, or synovium—makes a slick liquid called the synovial fluid that lubricates the joint. In many forms of arthritis, the synovium becomes inflamed and thickened, producing extra fluid containing inflammatory cells. Under the right circumstances, these inflammatory cells can then attack and damage the cartilage and the bone underlying it.

Although scientists researching arthritis have come a long way toward understanding how joints work, we still don't know exactly what causes arthritis. Even so, prevention, early detection, and appropriate medical and surgical treatment can help most arthritis sufferers.

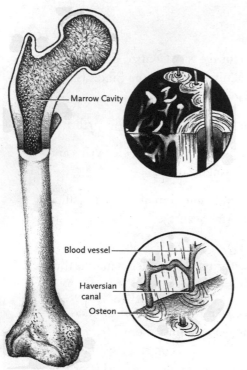

Bone is a living and dynamic organ.

Marrow Cavity

Blood vessel

Haversian canal

Osteon

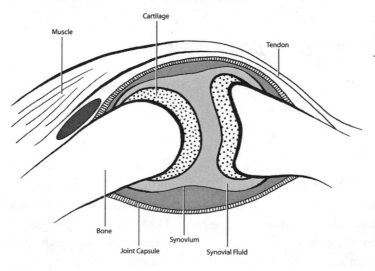

Muscle

Cartilage

Tendon

Anatomy of a normal joint.

Bone

Joint Capsule

Synovium

Synovial Fluid

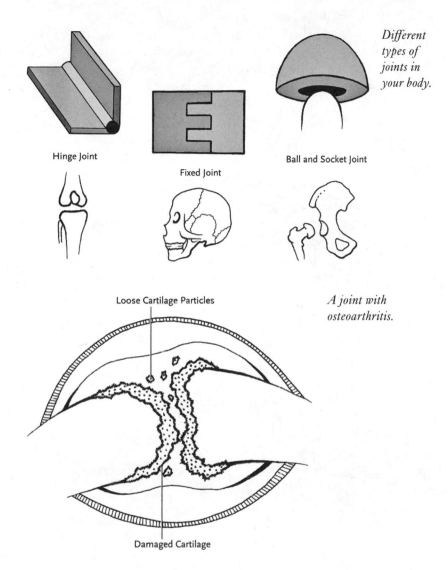

Different types of joints in your body.

Hinge Joint

Fixed Joint

Ball and Socket Joint

Loose Cartilage Particles

A joint with osteoarthritis.

Damaged Cartilage

COMMON FORMS OF ARTHRITIS: AN OVERVIEW

Osteoarthritis, the most common form of arthritis, occurs when joint cartilage breaks down, exposing bone ends and allowing them to rub together. The result can be pain, stiffness, loss of movement, and, sometimes, swelling. Osteoarthritis is most often found in the weight-bearing joints such as the hips, knees, ankles, and spine. There are many causes of osteoarthritis, including trauma, obesity, genetics, and other factors.

Rheumatoid arthritis is the second-most-common form of arthri-

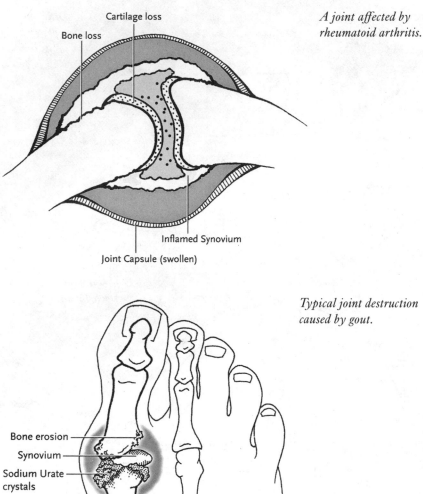

Bone loss

Cartilage loss

A joint affected by rheumatoid arthritis.

Inflamed Synovium

Joint Capsule (swollen)

Typical joint destruction caused by gout.

Bone erosion

Synovium

Sodium Urate crystals

tis, and it occurs when the immune system turns against the body. The faulty immune system causes inflammation and swelling that begins in the joint lining and spreads to the cartilage and the bone. Rheumatoid arthritis tends to affect joints symmetrically — in other words, it tends to affect the same joint on both sides of the body (for example, both hands or both wrists).

Gout is caused by the buildup of uric acid, which forms crystals that deposit in the joint. These needlelike crystals cause inflammation

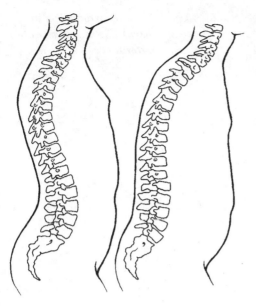

Ankylosing spondylitis leads to loss of normal spine curvature.

leading to severe pain and are most commonly found in the knees, the wrists, and the big toe. Heredity, diet, and certain drugs may cause or exacerbate gout.

Pseudogout occurs when calcium crystals deposit within joints. The symptoms are similar to those of gout, but, unlike gout, pseudogout is not caused or exacerbated by dietary habits.

Ankylosing spondylitis is a chronic inflammation of the spine that causes the vertebrae to eventually fuse together, giving the spine a very rigid appearance. Although the cause is unknown, genetics is thought to play a large role.

Infectious arthritis occurs when bacteria, viruses, or fungi enter the body, settle in the joints, and cause fever, inflammation, and joint destruction.

Juvenile arthritis encompasses different kinds of arthritis that strike children under the age of sixteen, the most common of which is juvenile rheumatoid arthritis. Pain or swelling in the shoulders, elbows, knees, ankles, or toes; chills; a reappearing fever; and sometimes a body rash are many of the common symptoms. The cause remains unknown.

Psoriatic arthritis occurs in conjunction with the inherited skin condition psoriasis, which causes scaly, red, rough patches on the neck, elbows, and knees. Psoriatic arthritis often afflicts the joints of the fingers and toes, causing the digits to swell.

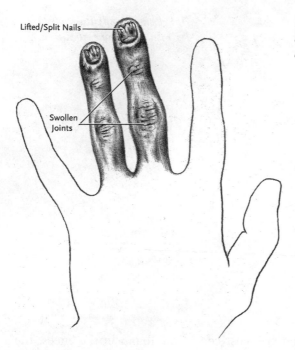

Lifted/Split Nails

Swollen Joints

Typical appearance of a hand afflicted with psoriatic arthritis.

THE MANY CAUSES OF JOINT PAIN

Whether arthritis has developed because of genetic factors or, far more commonly, torn cartilage, sprains, and dislocations, joint pain is a condition that can be most effectively treated—and prevented—when its causes are understood.

Osteoarthritis

As mentioned earlier, osteoarthritis, which is sometimes called degenerative arthritis or degenerative joint disease, is the result of the breakdown of cartilage inside the joint. When the cartilage that cushions bone ends no longer does its job, the bone ends can't slide easily across each other within the joint. That's when the pain and stiffness begin.

What Is Cartilage?

Three different types of cartilage are found in the body. The smooth articular, or hyaline, cartilage covers joint surfaces. Its function is to provide a low-friction surface to help the joint withstand the stress and strain that occurs with daily weight-bearing activities such as walking, stair climbing, and exercise. The ultrastrong fibrocartilage is found in the knee and

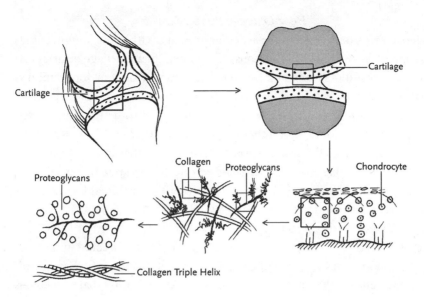

Our joints are complex structures that on a microscopic level involve the intricate interaction of cells (chondrocytes), water, collagen, and various proteins such as proteoglycans.

within the vertebral disks and is used to help connect bones. And the stiff but soft elastic cartilage, which is used to keep open passageways in the body, is found in such places as the ear canals and the throat.

Cartilage is made up of four ingredients:

1. Water. Most of cartilage, 65–85 percent, is water, which lubricates the joints, cushions bones, and absorbs shock.

2. Collagen. The joint gains elasticity and the ability to be a shock absorber from collagen, a connective tissue that is arranged in a meshlike framework and holds bones and muscles together.

3. Proteoglycans. The large molecules called proteoglycans embed themselves securely into the collagen mesh and soak up water like a sponge (they can also release water). The proteoglycans allow cartilage to expand and contract, molding to the shape of the joint as the pressure within the joint capsule changes with activity.

4. Chondrocytes. The important chondrocyte cells break down and get rid of old proteoglycan and collagen molecules, forming new ones to take their place.

How Osteoarthritis Starts

Osteoarthritis occurs when the articular cartilage within the joint becomes disrupted (from a variety of reasons). These articular cartilage injuries can occur as a result of a sudden injury (such as a car accident or sports injury) or from ordinary wear and tear. Depending on the extent of the damage and the location of the injury, articular cartilage can sometimes heal itself, but complete restoration is difficult because articular cartilage has no direct blood supply. (Perhaps surprisingly, an injury that involves the bone beneath the cartilage has a better chance of healing despite being a deeper injury, because the underlying bone will provide some blood for the cartilage to renourish and possibly heal itself.)

Osteoarthritis generally develops in three stages. First, there is a loss of cartilage or an injury to the cartilage within the affected joint. Second, the body tries to repair the cartilage and is unsuccessful; and third, the bone beneath the cartilage becomes sclerotic, meaning that it becomes abnormally thickened or hardened.

Once your cartilage is damaged, the tissue that is laid down to try to repair the injury is always biomechanically inferior to articular cartilage. In addition, injured cartilage will occasionally lay down bone instead of cartilage in its attempt to heal itself, forming an irregular surface that doesn't glide smoothly against the cartilage on the opposing bone end. Sometimes, too, the cartilage doesn't try to repair itself at all. Pieces of loose cartilage and/or bone may break off and float freely around the joint (these are called loose bodies, or joint mice, and can sometimes cause the joint to lock). Now the bone ends are no longer well padded, and they start to rub against each other and begin to develop bony spurs (osteophytes). The joint space narrows, and the entire shape of the joint begins to change. All this from a little damaged cartilage.

Signs and Symptoms of Osteoarthritis

How do you know whether the joint pain you're suffering from is the result of osteoarthritis? Most of those with the disease have at least one of the following symptoms:

> JOINT PAIN. Most people experience joint pain as a deep-seated ache. The feeling is different from a muscular ache and may come and go according to changes in the weather. People sometimes say, "I can feel it in my bones when it's going to rain." The pain is

usually worse with activity and better with rest, although the pain can become more constant in later stages.

STIFFNESS. Stiff joints, limited range of motion, and, in later stages, joints that don't move at all are all signs of osteoarthritis. Morning stiffness is present but usually lasts less than thirty minutes.

SWELLING. Although swelling does not always occur with osteoarthritis, some joints do swell in response to the cartilage damage found in osteoarthritis. The finger joints and the knees are most often affected.

BONY GROWTHS ON THE FINGERS. Bony lumps, either at the ends of the fingers (called Heberden's nodes) or on the middle joint of the fingers (called Bouchard's nodes), are signs of osteoarthritis. These types of bony growths may be hereditary.

Causes of Osteoarthritis

When we don't know why cartilage deteriorates, we designate the problem as primary osteoarthritis, or osteoarthritis of unknown cause. Approximately 80–90 percent of individuals older than sixty-five suffer from primary osteoarthritis. Osteoarthritis of known cause, by contrast, is called secondary arthritis. This kind of arthritis typically afflicts younger individuals, and it can occur after an injury, infection, or other trauma to the cartilage.

The cause of primary osteoarthritis remains unknown. Although scientists aren't sure why, the collagen mesh of the cartilage becomes scrambled; it weakens and can't hold its structure. The proteoglycans lose their place in the collagen mesh, and, as they float off into the joint fluid, they take their water-retaining abilities with them. The cartilage is left high and dry; it thins and may even crack. At the same time, the newly freed proteoglycans draw excess fluid into the joint capsule, causing swelling.

Some ideas about what causes primary arthritis are emerging among experts:

- The chondrocytes that are responsible for creating enzymes that break down and replace the collagen and proteoglycan molecules may become inefficient. In healthy cartilage, the amount of breaking-down enzymes is equal to the amount of building-up enzymes. An overabundance of destructive enzymes would lead to weakened collagen and a lack of proteoglycans.

• In an almost opposite scenario, the chondrocytes may go wild and start making too many proteoglycan and collagen molecules. Ironically, the excess proteoglycan and collagen molecules that are made end up pulling extra fluid into the joint, flooding it and washing away most of the chondrocytes. The cartilage, then, is left without any cartilage-producing molecules.

• Conditions that lead to cartilage loss and potentially secondary osteoarthritis include injury, obesity, crystal deposits, infection, congenital abnormalities (abnormalities present at birth), or joint surgery. In particular:

JOINT INJURY. Once a joint has been injured, it is more likely to develop arthritis. If you have suffered a traumatic injury from an event such as a motor vehicle accident, have played rough-and-tumble sports, or have injured any of your joints in any way, you are more likely to develop osteoarthritis in the joints that were affected by those activities.

REPETITIVE MOTION INJURY (OVERUSE). Joints that are repeatedly stressed in the same way are more likely to experience cartilage breakdown than joints subjected to normal use. Ballet dancers, assembly line workers, baseball pitchers, carpenters, heavy laborers, and anyone else who overuses and stresses a joint or joints can suffer from cartilage breakdown in their overused joints.

DAMAGE TO THE END OF THE BONE. Usually the result of trauma or continual stress, a bone may chip or sustain small fractures. The body, in its attempt to repair the damage, may cause an overgrowth of bone in the injured area. The result is a bone end that is bumpy rather than smooth.

BONE DISEASE. A bone disorder such as Paget's disease may weaken the bone structure, making it more likely to fracture and develop bony overgrowth.

CARRYING TOO MUCH BODY WEIGHT. The heavier you are, the more stress your knees, hips, and ankles must bear. Osteoarthritis of the knee has been linked to excess body weight. That's not surprising considering that every time you take a walking step the stress on your knee is roughly equivalent to three times your body weight, and, when you run, that figure is increased to about ten times your body weight.

Contributing Risk Factors for Osteoarthritis

Although osteoarthritis affects millions of Americans, not everyone suffers from it. Some people grow old with joints unaffected by pain, stiffness, or other symptoms, whereas others are hobbling around by the time they are thirty-five. Why does one person get osteoarthritis while another stays healthy? And how can you tell if you are susceptible to developing the disease?

In addition to the risk factors detailed earlier for secondary osteoarthritis, your chances of developing the disease vary according to:

YOUR RACE. The disorder is more prevalent in Native Americans than in the general population. Disease of the hip is seen less frequently in native Chinese than in Caucasians of similar age. In persons older than sixty-five years of age, osteoarthritis is more common in whites than in blacks.

YOUR AGE. Cartilage and other joint structures, like most bodily tissues, tend to degrade and become weaker over time. After decades of use, they start to wear out. Luckily, research has shown that osteoarthritis isn't inevitable as we age—just more likely.

YOUR SEX. In individuals older than fifty-five, the prevalence of osteoarthritis is higher among women than among men. In those younger than forty-five, however, the prevalence of osteoarthritis is higher among men. Women are especially susceptible to osteoarthritis in the distal interphalangeal joints (the finger joint closest to the fingernail). Osteoarthritis of the hip, by contrast, appears to occur more commonly in men than in women.

YOUR PARENTS. There appears to be a genetic component to osteoarthritis; in fact, one study concluded that genes were responsible for 50 percent of hip osteoarthritis cases. Osteoarthritis in the hands is also believed to be at least partially due to genetics. An inherited tendency toward defective cartilage or poorly structures joints can certainly put you on the road to osteoarthritis, although you won't necessarily develop it.

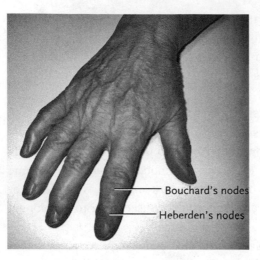

Typical findings associated with osteoarthritis of the hand.

Bouchard's nodes

Heberden's nodes

Diagnosing Osteoarthritis

Osteoarthritis is diagnosed mainly by detailed history and physical examination, because many common laboratory tests are not helpful in diagnosing the disease. For example, although osteoarthritis is quite common in people over age sixty-five, fewer than half of those who suffer from it—and generally only those with advanced cases of the disease—have symptoms visible via conventional X-rays. Magnetic resonance imaging is more sensitive, but in some cases direct visualization of the joint during surgery (arthroscopy) is the only way to know for sure whether osteoarthritis is the correct diagnosis.

To further aid in the diagnosis of osteoarthritis in particular joints, the American College of Rheumatology has come up with two sets of criteria for such a diagnosis:

> FOR THE KNEE: The patient has knee pain and osteophytes, and is either (1) over age fifty, (2) suffering from stiffness of the knee joint for more than thirty minutes a day, or (3) experiencing crepitus (crunchiness in the joint).

> FOR THE HIP: The patient is having hip pain and has two of the following diagnostic features: X-ray evidence of osteophytes, X-ray evidence of joint narrowing, and an erythrocyte sedimentation rate (ESR) of less than twenty. ESR levels are typically high in patients suffering from autoimmune disease or infection, and these

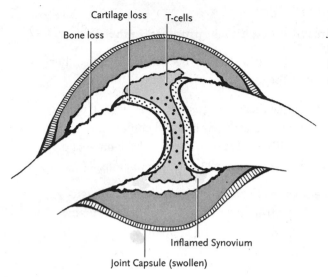

Cartilage loss   T-cells

Bone loss

Inflamed Synovium

Joint Capsule (swollen)

The mechanism of joint destruction and associated symptoms of rheumatoid arthritis.

processes need to be ruled out prior to diagnosing a patient with osteoarthritis.

Rheumatoid Arthritis

Rheumatoid arthritis is a case of the human body's good intentions gone awry. Your body is equipped with a very effective immune system that fights off bacteria and other foreign bodies. Specialized immune cells attack these invaders, surround them, paralyze them, and destroy them. A strong, intact immune system is absolutely essential to your survival— without it, you would quickly be overcome by infections and disease. But with rheumatoid arthritis, your immune system goes haywire and starts attacking your body's own tissues. That is, when you have rheumatoid arthritis, your own immune system (T cells) attacks the tissues that cushion and line your joints, eventually causing entire joints to deteriorate. Rheumatoid arthritis can affect any joint in the body. But it usually affects the small joints in the hands and feet before any of the larger joints, such as hips or knees.

Although the condition can develop at any age, rheumatoid arthritis is most likely to emerge between the ages of twenty and forty-five. It seems that the older you are when rheumatoid arthritis first strikes, the milder your case is likely to be. Rarely, children under the age of sixteen can develop a form of rheumatoid arthritis known as juvenile rheumatoid

---

Notable Individuals with Rheumatoid Arthritis

- Actress Lucille Ball, whose left leg became shorter than her right as a result of the disease.

- Impressionist painter Pierre-Auguste Renoir, who struggled with painful rheumatoid arthritis but still completed artworks infused with joy. He is thought to have once said about his art, "The pain passes but the joy remains."

- The Roman emperor Diocletian, who exempted citizens with severe arthritis from paying taxes, no doubt realizing that the disease itself can be taxing enough.

---

arthritis, or Still's disease. Rheumatoid arthritis afflicts all ethnic groups, yet despite some very serious consequences many people with rheumatoid arthritis live long, successful lives. Just remember that early treatment can make a big difference, so don't wait to see a doctor.

The Body Becomes Its Own Worst Enemy

For reasons that aren't completely understood, in rheumatoid arthritis the white blood cells of the immune system attack the joint lining (synovial membrane) as if it were a foreign object. Pain, loss of movement, and joint destruction are the unhappy results. After the immune system goes to work on the joint lining,

1. The assaulted membrane becomes inflamed and painful, the entire joint capsule swells, and the synovial cells start to grow and divide in an abnormal way.

2. The now abnormal synovial cells start to invade the surrounding tissue—mostly the bone and cartilage.

3. The joint space begins to narrow, and the joint's supporting structures become weak. At the same time, the cells that trigger inflammation release enzymes that eat away at the bone and cartilage, causing joint erosion and scarring.

4. The joint itself deteriorates, eventually becoming deformed.

Symptoms of Rheumatoid Arthritis

Although the symptoms of rheumatoid arthritis vary, most people experience one or more of the following:

- Pain, warmth, redness, swelling, or tightness in a joint

- Swelling of three or more joints for six or more weeks

- Joints affected in a symmetrical pattern (for example, both knees)

- Joint pain or stiffness lasting longer than an hour upon arising in the morning or after prolonged inactivity

- Pea-shaped bumps under the skin (called rheumatoid nodules), especially on pressure points like the elbows or the feet. In bedridden patients, they may also occur at the base of the scalp or on the back hip area

- Evidence of joint erosion on an X-ray

- Loss of mobility

- General soreness, aching, or stiffness

- A general "sick" feeling (malaise)

- Fatigue and weakness

- Periodic low-grade fever and/or sweating

- Difficulty sleeping

- Anemia (low blood count)

Rarely, rheumatoid arthritis causes problems with other parts of the body. These problems may include inflammation of the blood vessels (vasculitis), inflammation of the linings of the lung or the heart, and dryness of the eyes and mouth (Sjogren's syndrome).

Possible Causes of Rheumatoid Arthritis

The truth is that nobody really knows what causes rheumatoid arthritis, although some believe it is linked to a defect in the immune system. Many people with the disease have a particular genetic marker—HLA-DR4— although not everyone with this gene ends up with rheumatoid arthritis (and not everyone with rheumatoid arthritis has this gene). Most scientists currently believe that HLA-DR4 is only one of several genes that predispose someone to developing the disease.

Some researchers believe that rheumatoid arthritis may be triggered by a virus or bacteria that causes the immune system to wrongly attack the lining of the joints (perhaps because the virus houses molecules that, to the immune system, look similar to molecules within the joint). Unfortunately, this infectious agent has yet to be found. Other researchers believe that hormones may be involved in the development of rheumatoid arthritis. Women are more likely than men to develop rheumatoid arthritis, suggesting a possible link to estrogen.

Diagnosing Rheumatoid Arthritis

There is no single test that can diagnose rheumatoid arthritis. Instead, the diagnosis is typically made by a physician based on:

- A full medical history, including any family history of rheumatoid arthritis

- Discussion of current symptoms

- A physical examination of the joints and skin, as well as tests of reflexes and muscle strength

- X rays

- Blood tests. Two blood tests commonly performed to assist in the diagnosis of rheumatoid arthritis are a screen for rheumatoid factor (or RhF), a protein produced by the immune system that is present in as many as 80 percent of people with rheumatoid arthritis, and an erythrocyte sedimentation rate (an elevated ESR usually indicates the presence of inflammation somewhere in the body).

OTHER COMMON CAUSES OF JOINT PAIN

Many people who are active in sports find themselves injured from time to time. Unfortunately, such injuries can reemerge decades later as pain in the parts of the joint called ligaments and tendons. While both add to our joint stability, each has a very specific role within the joint: ligaments attach bone to bone, whereas tendons attach muscle to bone. The most common types of joint injuries are ligament sprains, bone bruises or contusions, cartilage tears, bony dislocations, and fractures (broken bones).

Here we describe these injuries only briefly; later chapters will focus in depth on specific injuries to each joint.

Sprains

A sprain is an injury to a ligament. In a sprain, one or more ligaments is stretched or torn. Falling, twisting, or getting hit can force a joint out of its normal position, causing ligaments around the joint to stretch or tear. Sprains happen most often in the ankle.

The usual signs and symptoms of a sprain are pain, swelling, bruising, and not being able to move or use a joint. Sometimes people feel a pop or tear when the injury happens. A sprain can be mild, moderate, or severe. Most sprains can be treated effectively with rest, ice, compression, and elevation (RICE), although as we explain in later chapters, certain severe, recurrent tears may require a trip to the operating room for repair.

Strains

A strain occurs when a muscle or a tendon is stretched or torn after being twisted or pulled. Strains can happen suddenly or develop over a period of time. Acute strains are usually caused by lifting objects the wrong way or by overstressing muscles; chronic strains are usually caused by moving the muscles and tendons the same way over and over. Muscles that are most commonly strained are the back muscles and the hamstring muscles in the back of the thigh. A strain can cause pain, muscle spasms, muscle weakness, swelling, cramping, and difficulty in moving the muscle.

Torn Cartilage

Torn cartilage is frequently seen around or in the knee in sports that create sudden twisting motions such as football, basketball, or tennis. Treatment usually involves physical therapy if the injury is minor or, if the injury is more severe, surgery to remove the torn cartilage pieces. This intervention is important because mature cartilage generally does not heal itself well; consequently, torn cartilage can and often does lead to osteoarthritis.

Dislocations

Dislocations occur when injuries push the bones out of their normal positions within the joint. Treatment of bony dislocations involves the realignment of the bones by a medical professional. These types of injuries can

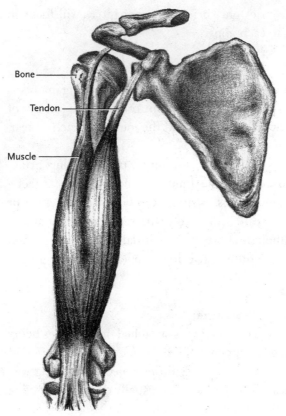

Relationship between bone, tendon, and muscle.

Bone

Tendon

Muscle

have multiple associated injuries including fractures and ligament ruptures as well as nerve and vessel injuries. The most frequently dislocated
joint is the finger. Whereas finger dislocations rarely produce catastrophic
consequences, shoulder, elbow, hip, knee, or ankle dislocations can cause
lifelong problems.

It can be difficult to tell a broken bone from a dislocated bone. In
either case, get medical help right away. While you're waiting for medical
attention:

DON'T MOVE THE JOINT. Splint or sling the affected joint in its
current position. Don't try to move a dislocated joint or force it
back into place. This can damage the joint and its surrounding
muscles, ligaments, nerves, and/or blood vessels.

ICE THE INJURED JOINT. Applying ice to the injured joint can help
reduce pain and swelling by controlling internal bleeding and the
buildup of fluids in and around it.

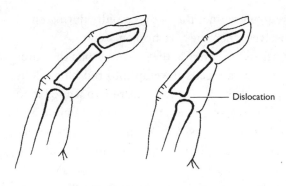

With a dislocation, there is a loss of the normal relationship between bone ends.

Dislocation

Treatment of the dislocation depends on the severity of the injury and where it occurred. Your doctor may try some gentle maneuvers to help your bones back into position—a process called reduction. Depending on the amount of pain and swelling, you may need a local anesthetic or even a general anesthetic to ease the pain before your bones can be manipulated in this way.

After your bones are back in place, any severe pain should resolve. Your doctor may immobilize your joint with a splint or sling for several weeks. How long you wear the splint or sling depends on the nature of your dislocation and where it occurred. Your doctor may also prescribe a pain reliever or a muscle relaxant.

After your splint or sling is removed, you will begin a rehabilitation program designed to restore gradually your joint's range of motion and strength. Avoid strenuous activity with your injured joint until it has regained full movement and normal strength and stability. If you have experienced a generally simple dislocation (that is, one without major nerve or tissue damage), your joint likely will return to a near- or fully normal condition. But trying to come back too soon from such an injury may cause you to reinjure the joint.

In rare cases, you may need surgery for a dislocation if your blood vessels or nerves are damaged or if your doctor can't manipulate your dislocated bones back into their correct positions. Surgery may also be necessary if you have weak joints or ligaments and tend to have recurring dislocations.

Fractures

Fractures are broken bones. To understand why bones break, it helps to know what bones do and what they are made of. The bones of the body form the human frame, or skeleton, which supports and protects the softer parts of the body. Bones are living tissue; they grow rapidly during one's early years and repair themselves when they are broken.

Bones have a center, called the marrow, that is softer than the outer part of the bone. Some bone marrow cells develop into red blood cells that carry oxygen to all parts of the body; others mature into white blood cells that help fight disease. Bones also contain the minerals calcium and phosphorus, which are combined in a crystal-like or latticework structure. Because of their unique structure, bones can bear large amounts of weight.

Fractures can occur in a variety of ways, but there are three common causes:

TRAUMA. A fall, a motor vehicle accident, or a tackle during a football game can all result in fractures.

OSTEOPOROSIS. Osteoporosis is a bone disease that results in the "thinning" of the bone. The bones become fragile and break easily.

OVERUSE. Fractures from overuse (stress fractures) are common among athletes.

Most of the time you will know immediately if you've broken a bone. You may hear a snap or cracking sound, and the area around the fracture will be tender and swollen. A limb may be deformed, or a part of the bone may pierce the skin. Doctors usually use an X-ray to verify the diagnosis. Stress fractures are more difficult than other fractures to diagnose, because they may not immediately appear on an X-ray, but they may cause pain, tenderness, or mild swelling.

When you arrive at the doctor's office or hospital with a possible fracture, the physician in charge will determine first whether you have a closed, or simple, fracture, in which the bone is broken, but the skin surrounding it is not destroyed; or an open (sometimes called "compound") fracture. In an open fracture, the skin may be pierced by the bone or it may have been broken open by a blow at the time of the fracture. The bone may or may not be visible in the wound.

There are different kinds of compound fractures, including transverse fracture, in which the fracture is at right angles to the long axis of the bone; greenstick fracture, where the fracture is on one side of the bone, causing a bend on the other side of the bone (more common in children);

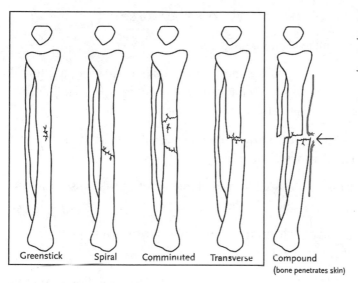

Greenstick   Spiral   Comminuted   Transverse   Compound
(bone penetrates skin)

A variety of fracture types are possible, from minor (Greenstick) to severe (compound).

and comminuted fracture, in which the fracture has resulted in three or more bone fragments.

As soon as a fracture occurs, the body acts to protect the injured area, forming a protective blood clot and callus (fibrous tissue). New "threads" of bone cells start to grow on both sides of the fracture line and grow toward each other. After the fracture is closed the callus is absorbed.

Doctors use many devices to hold a fracture in the correct position while the bone is healing. External fixation methods include plaster and fiberglass casts, cast-braces, and splints, whereas internal fixation methods hold the broken pieces of bone in their proper position for healing with metal plates, pins, or screws.

Fractures take from several weeks to several months to heal, depending on the extent of the injury and how well you follow your doctor's advice. The pain usually stops long before the fracture is solid enough to handle the stresses of normal activity, so even after your cast or brace is removed, you may need to continue limiting your daily activities. Usually, by the time the bone is strong enough, the muscles, particularly in the case of a broken leg or arm, will be weak because they haven't been used. Your ligaments may feel "stiff" from not using them. Before those tissues will again perform their functions normally, you will need a period of rehabilitation that involves exercises and gradually increasing activity.

MAIN POINTS TO REMEMBER:

- There are many forms of arthritis.

- A joint is made up of the ends of two bones, cartilage that lines the ends of the bones, a joint capsule containing synovial fluid, and ligaments and tendons that support the joint.

- Osteoarthritis is the most common cause of arthritis, followed by rheumatoid arthritis and gout.

- Osteoarthritis is caused by a combination of age, overuse of joints, injury, genetics, and infection.

- Genetics play a role in some forms of arthritis, namely rheumatoid arthritis and ankylosing spondylitis.

- Although the cause of primary osteoarthritis is unknown, avoiding traumatic joint injuries can prevent secondary osteoarthritis.

- Rheumatoid arthritis occurs when the body's immune system goes awry and starts attacking the synovial lining of its own joints.

- Sprains, strains, dislocations, torn cartilage, and fractures can occur with any joint.

PART ONE

Where Joint Pain Occurs

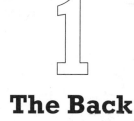

The Back

BACK PAIN IS A HEALTH concern for millions of people, with eight of ten people experiencing back pain at some point in their lives. In 2002 alone, there were more than thirty million visits to physician's offices because of back pain.

The back is composed of bones, muscles, ligaments, tendons, and cartilage that run from the neck to the pelvis. The vertebrae are stacked on top of each other and form a spinal column that supports the upper body's weight and protects the spinal cord. The spinal cord is part of the central nervous system that helps carry signals to control your body's movements and sensations; it originates at the base of the brain and extends in the adult to just below the ribs. Nerves enter and exit the spinal cord through spaces between each vertebrae; the space between the vertebrae is maintained by round, spongy pads of cartilage called intervertebral disks. These disks act like shock absorbers while ligaments and tendons hold the vertebrae in place and attach muscles to the spinal column.

From the skull down, the spine has four regions:

- seven cervical, or neck, vertebrae (C1–C7),
- twelve thoracic, or upper back, vertebrae (T1–T12),
- five lumbar, or lower back, vertebrae (L1–L5), and the
- sacrum and coccyx, the back bones we sit on.

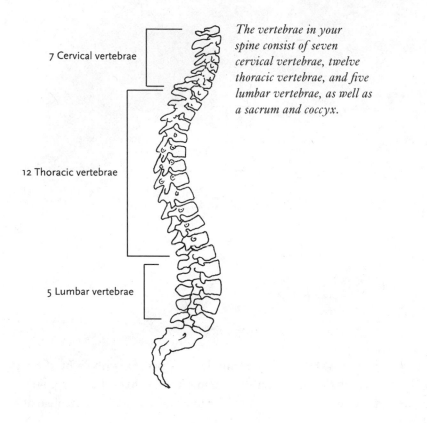

7 Cervical vertebrae

12 Thoracic vertebrae

5 Lumbar vertebrae

The vertebrae in your spine consist of seven cervical vertebrae, twelve thoracic vertebrae, and five lumbar vertebrae, as well as a sacrum and coccyx.

SPINAL STENOSIS

Spinal stenosis affects between 250,000 and 500,000 people in the United States alone. In spinal stenosis, the spinal canal becomes narrow and pinches the spinal cord nerves. About three-quarters of the patients who suffer from spinal stenosis are affected in their lumbar spine, although stenosis can also affect the upper (or cervical) spine. In most instances of lumbar stenosis the sciatic nerve is compressed, causing pain that runs down the buttocks.

Causes

There are many causes of spinal stenosis. The most common are

- Aging. As you age, bone spurs can develop on the vertebrae, compressing the spinal canal and/or nerve roots. Ligaments around the spine will thicken with age as well, and the cushioning disks between the vertebrae will start to deteriorate, fragment, and dry out.

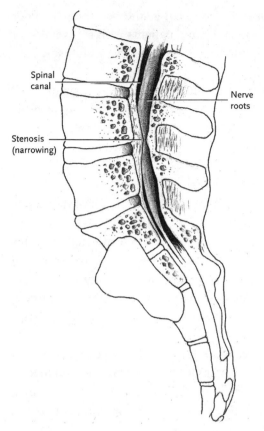

Spinal canal

Nerve roots

Stenosis (narrowing)

In spinal stenosis, the spinal canal is narrowed due to an overgrowth of bone and soft tissue.

- Heredity. Some people are born with a narrower spinal canal and are at increased risk of spinal stenosis.

- Trauma. Accidents and trauma during your life may result in spinal fractures that can result in acute or slowly progressive nerve root or spinal compression.

Symptoms

If you have spinal stenosis, you will most likely experience pain or cramping in your legs when you walk or stand for long periods, as a result of the compression of the nerves in the lower spine. Bending forward tends to ease the pain, because flexing the spine opens up more space for, and takes some pressure off, the nerves.

You may also experience a loss of balance or clumsiness if pressure on the spinal cord affects the nerves that control your balance.

Cervical (neck) stenosis can cause pain in the neck and shoulder region that may extend to the arm and hand; patients with this version of spinal stenosis may also suffer headaches, muscle weakness, clumsiness, or decreased sensation.

Loss of bowel or bladder function, or "cauda equina syndrome," can also be an issue in severe cases of stenosis, when the nerves to the bladder or bowel may be compressed. Anyone with partial or complete urinary or fecal incontinence should seek immediate medical attention.

Diagnosis

Spinal stenosis can be difficult to diagnose because of its very gradual onset and because many people who develop the condition have no history of back problems or trauma. In addition, many people affected with this condition also suffer from diabetes, cardiovascular disease, or peripheral vascular disease—diseases that can produce similar symptoms. Often, unusual leg symptoms such as pain or numbness around one's buttocks are clues to spinal stenosis, but many other diseases have similar symptoms.

X-rays, MRIs, and CT scans are often needed to diagnose spinal stenosis definitively. In addition your spine specialist may order a myelogram (an X-ray taken after a special fluid is injected into the spine), which offers a clearer, more detailed view of the bones and soft tissues involved.

Nonsurgical Treatments

Nonsurgical recommendations for treating spinal stenosis include:

- Changes in posture, for example leaning slightly forward while walking to flex the spine, or lying down at night with knees drawn up to your chest

- Nonsteroidal anti-inflammatory drugs (NSAIDs)

- Rest

- Low-impact aerobic activities, such as bicycling or water aerobics

- Weight loss, to relieve the load on the spine

- A lumbar brace

- Epidural steroid injections

Surgical Treatments

The goal of surgery is to relieve pressure on the spinal cord so that your symptoms will ease. Muscle atrophy can be difficult to reverse, however, and in fact is often permanent. Moreover, although back surgery can relieve pain, it's no cure-all. Recovery can take weeks or months and may require long-term physical therapy. In addition, surgery won't stop the degenerative process and symptoms may return—sometimes within just a few years.

Common surgical procedures include:

DECOMPRESSIVE LAMINECTOMY. In this surgery the lamina—the bone that makes up the back of the spinal canal—is removed to create more space for the nerves and to allow access to bone spurs or ruptured disks that may need to be removed during surgery. The surgery itself is often performed through a single incision in the back (open surgery). Risks related to laminectomy include bleeding, infection, nerve damage, a tear in the membrane (dura) that covers the spinal cord, and impaired bowel function (thankfully, this side effect is usually transient).

FUSION. Fusion, which is often performed along with a laminectomy, involves connecting two or more vertebral bones in the spine to prevent the vertebrae from slipping over one another.

General Tips for Prevention

Although it is difficult to prevent degenerative changes in your back, the following steps can help keep your back in good shape:

EXERCISE REGULARLY. Exercise can help you maintain your ideal body weight, which decreases the load on the spine; it can also ensure that you will maintain strength and flexibility in your spine. In addition, strengthening your back, leg, arm, and abdominal muscles can take stress off your back. When considering an exercise program, consult with your doctor first for ideas on how to find the right exercises for you. You will probably want to combine aerobic activities such as walking and biking with weight training and stretching. And be sure to stretch gently before you exercise to help reduce wear and tear on your back.

MAINTAIN APPROPRIATE BODY MECHANICS. Adopt appropriate techniques for sitting, standing, lifting heavy objects, and sleep-

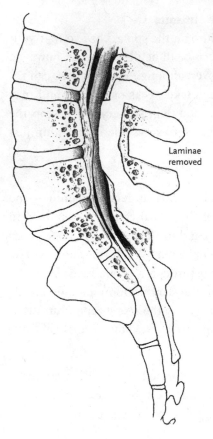

During laminectomy, the laminae are removed to relieve pressure on the spinal cord.

Laminae removed

ing. For example, when lifting be careful to bend your knees so that your arms are level with the object being lifted; when you lift something heavy, avoid lifting it overhead. Sit in a chair that supports your lower back, particularly when you are sitting for long periods of time—if necessary, place a pillow against your lower back to maintain its normal curve. And, while you are driving, adjust your seat to keep your knees and hips level, and be sure to take frequent breaks so you can walk and stretch.

SCOLIOSIS

Scoliosis, which afflicts about 2 percent of the population, is a disorder that slowly causes a sideways S- or C-shaped curve of the spine. Although people of any age, ethnicity, or sex can suffer from scoliosis, the most com-

Does Posture Matter?

It's true: good posture (standing up straight, sitting straight, and lifting with your back straight) can help your back. So bend your knees and hips when you lift something, and keep your back straight. When you hold an object, carry it close to your body. When you stand for prolonged periods, elevate one foot for a while (place it on a stool or step). And when you sit for long stretches, elevate your feet on a stool so your knees are higher than your hips. These measures decrease pressure on your disk and help to prevent injury.

mon type, idiopathic scoliosis, afflicts children between the ages of ten and the early teenage years.

Causes

The cause of scoliosis is unknown. When it emerges in adulthood, it is usually thought to be the result of either the progression of an undiagnosed childhood scoliosis or age-related degenerative changes of the spine. Both the adult and child forms seem to run in families. Other factors that contribute to spine curvature seem to be:

- Sex. Girls have a higher risk of curve progression than boys.

- Age. Younger children with scoliosis are at greater risk of curve progression than are older children.

- Angle of the curve at time of diagnosis. The more the back is curved, the more likely the disease is to progress.

- Location. Scoliosis affecting the upper spine (cervical and thoracic areas) is more likely to progress than scoliosis affecting the mid- to lower spine.

- Spinal problems at birth. Children who have scoliosis at birth may experience rapid advancement of their disease.

Signs of scoliosis include: uneven shoulders, prominent shoulder blades, uneven leg lengths, uneven waist, uneven hip elevation (one hip higher

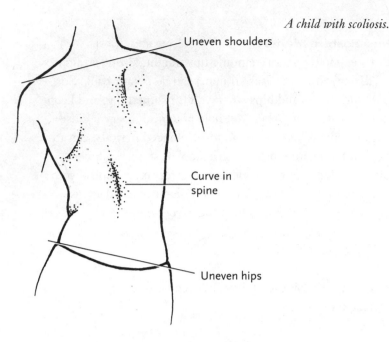

A child with scoliosis.

Uneven shoulders

Curve in
spine

Uneven hips

than the other), and leaning to one side. Because the onset of scoliosis is gradual and typically painless, a significant curvature can develop without the parent or child even noticing it. Early detection is important to prevent the curve from progressing, so examine your child carefully if you notice any signs of curvature—and if you do detect it, see a doctor for further advice. It is especially important to examine the spine regularly if there is a family history of scoliosis.

Diagnosis

In addition to taking a careful medical and genetic history and examining your spine, your doctor will most likely X-ray the spine to help determine whether you have scoliosis. The X-ray will determine the degree of curvature in addition to its location, shape, and pattern.

Treatments

Treatment for scoliosis depends on many factors. Your doctor will consider your age, the degree and type of curvature, and the potential for further curve progression. Depending on the diagnosis, your physician may recommend observation, bracing, or surgery. Observation is frequently the chosen course for those children who are still growing and who have spinal curves that are less than 25 degrees. A physician should examine these children every four to six months. And in those cases where it is needed, a brace can effectively slow curve progression, although this is not a favorite treatment among image-conscious adolescent girls and boys.

Surgery is generally recommended if a curve is progressing rapidly, if it is more than 45 degrees, or if it makes the back look deformed. Surgery usually involves fusing the bones of the spine together with the use of metal rods or other devices.

It is essential to monitor and treat scoliosis because, if left untreated, serious complications can occur. For example, severe scoliosis—a curve greater than 70 degrees—may cause the rib cage to press against the lungs and make breathing difficult. (In very severe scoliosis—a curve greater than 100 degrees—the lungs and heart may even become permanently deformed or damaged due to compression.) And adults who had scoliosis as children are more likely to suffer from chronic back pain.

Although sometimes essential, bracing during childhood and the teenage years may cause feelings of social isolation and lowered self-esteem. If you are a parent of a child wearing a brace, be ready to support your child emotionally during this difficult stage and be sure to seek a second opinion from a physician regarding whether bracing is the best alternative for your child's condition.

Prevention

Scoliosis does not seem to be a preventable disease. In particular, exercise programs have not been shown to slow the progression of scoliosis. Other ineffective preventative treatments include chiropractic therapy, electrical stimulation, and nutritional supplementation.

LOWER BACK PAIN

If your back aches, you're not alone. Four of five adults experience at least one attack of back pain during their lifetime; men and women are equally affected. The annual cost in terms of lost productivity, medical expenses, and workers' compensation benefits from back pain runs into the tens of billions of dollars in the United States alone.

Causes

The lower back (lumbar spine) is made up of five vertebrae; the lumbar disks between these vertebrae function as shock absorbers and allow for motion of the lumbar spine, while the spinal canal sits behind these disks.

Lower back pain may be a reflection of irritation in the nerves or muscles, or bone disease. Although most low back pain is caused by an injury, it can also be caused by a wide range of diseases, including arthritis or disk disease, osteoporosis, viral infections, or congenital spine disorders. Additional risk factors include smoking, obesity, poor posture, occupations that involve heavy lifting or other activities that can strain the back, genetics, and inadequate exercise.

Bone strength, as well as muscle elasticity and tone, tend to diminish with age; the disks also lose fluid, height, and flexibility. For this reason the risk of experiencing low back pain from disk disease or spinal degeneration increases with age (although most attacks occur between the ages of thirty and fifty). In the case of an injury, too, scar tissue created when the injured back heals itself is not as strong or as flexible as normal tissue. Pain with fever or loss of bowel or bladder control, pain when coughing, and progressive weakness in the legs may indicate a pinched nerve or other more serious condition. Diabetics sometimes experience severe back pain or pain radiating down the leg from neuropathy (nerve damage from the diabetes).

Specific medical conditions that may cause low back pain and require treatment include:

Bulging disk (also called protruding, herniated, or ruptured disk);

Spinal degeneration from disk wear and tear. This syndrome can lead to a narrowing of the spinal canal. If you have spinal degeneration, you may experience stiffness in the back upon awakening or feel pain after walking or standing for prolonged periods;

Spinal stenosis;

Osteoporosis;

Skeletal irregularities, such as scoliosis; kyphosis, a condition often seen in elderly women in which the upper back is severely rounded; lordosis, an abnormally accentuated arch in the lower back; or spondylitis, in which chronic back pain and stiffness are caused by a severe infection or inflammation of the spinal joints;

Fibromyalgia, a poorly understood chronic disorder characterized by musculoskeletal pain, fatigue, and multiple "tender points," particularly in the neck, spine, shoulders, and hips. Fibromyalgia sufferers may also experience poor sleep, morning stiffness, depression, and anxiety.

Symptoms

Most back pain sufferers experience an increase in pain when they bend over to pick something up; there may also be accompanying leg pain. The pain is most common in the back or outer part of the thigh and can travel all the way down to the foot (pain that goes to the foot is called sciatica because it follows the course of the sciatic nerve). Most acute episodes of back pain cause severe pain for up to a week with gradual improvement; by two to four weeks after onset the pain is often much improved. Most people find that a lying down position is least painful; most are able to rest at night without severe discomfort. Some get relief from arching backward (extending the back).

You should see a doctor immediately if your back pain:

- Is constant or severe, especially at night

- Spreads down one or both legs for longer than four to six weeks

- Causes new bowel or bladder problems

- Causes weakness, numbness, or tingling in one or both legs

- Is associated with abdominal pain or pulsation (throbbing)

- Is caused by a fall or blow to your back

- Is associated with unexplained or significant weight loss

Diagnosis

After obtaining your medical history, your doctor will check for evidence of nerve problems by evaluating your muscle strength, sensation, and reflexes. He or she may ask you to move your spine to see how limited your motion is. Traditional X-rays usually do not show abnormalities in patients with acute back pain and are not commonly ordered unless the pain does not improve for more than six weeks or there is evidence of more severe problems.

A history of cancer, significant trauma (for example, from a motor vehicle accident), or signs of active infection (fevers or chills) warrant the use of further imaging tests such as MRI or CT scans; significant weakness should also prompt immediate further imaging. If the patient is having trouble controlling urination or bowel habits, the doctor will usually also order X-rays and other studies.

Nonsurgical Treatments

Most lower back pain can be treated with activity modification, analgesics, exercise, and a prevention program. The basics of an initial conservative therapy include:

BED REST. Although it feels better initially than moving around, bed rest is not recommended for more than one or two days because recent studies suggest that prolonged bed rest may make back pain worse and lead to depression, decreased muscle tone, deconditioning, and blood clots. When in bed, patients should lie on one side with a pillow between their knees for maximum comfort;

ICE AND/OR HEAT. Although ice and heat have not been proven to heal lower back injuries, heat compresses are thought to help reduce pain, relax muscles, increase blood flow to the region, and allow improved mobility for some people. Cold compresses are also thought to decrease regional inflammation; patients should apply a cold pack to the tender area several times a day for up to twenty minutes at a time. As for whether heat or ice is better, we recommend that you try both and see which works best for you;

EXERCISE. Exercises that stretch and strengthen your back and abdominal muscles can help heal your low back pain. Activities that are healthy for the back include stretching exercises, swimming, walking, and movement therapy (which is designed to improve coordination and develop proper posture and muscle balance). In addition, it seems that yoga can play a role in the prevention of back pain. Your doctor may even recommend a "back school," an exercise program available in many communities and physical therapy centers that is meant to help you manage back pain and prevent it from recurring. Exercises learned there will help protect your back at home and at work. In addition, you might inquire about the McKenzie Method, a popular treatment program developed in the 1960s by Robin McKenzie, a physical therapist in New Zealand. McKenzie noted that extending the spine could provide significant pain relief to certain patients and allow them to return to their normal daily activities;

OVER-THE-COUNTER PAIN MEDICATIONS. Nonsteroidal anti-inflammatory drugs (NSAIDs), for example, can reduce lower back stiffness, swelling, and pain. And counter-irritants applied directly on the skin can stimulate the nerve endings in the skin, causing warm or cold sensations and dulling the pain (many of us can remember grandparents who used Ben-Gay on their back). Topical analgesics can also reduce inflammation and stimulate blood flow to ease pain;

PRESCRIPTION MEDICATIONS. Opioids such as codeine, oxycodone, and morphine are often prescribed to quell severe back pain; side effects can include drowsiness, impaired reaction time and judgment, and the potential for addiction. Indeed, many pain specialists are convinced that chronic use of opioids contributes to depression and can even worsen pain. In addition to opioids, antiseizure drugs can treat certain types of nerve pain and are sometimes prescribed for patients with back pain; antidepressants also have been shown to relieve pain by altering levels of brain chemicals to elevate mood and dull pain signals;

SPINAL MANIPULATION. In this hands-on approach, licensed specialists literally push the spinal structures into place in order to help restore back mobility.

Surgical Treatments

Surgery for low back pain should be considered or performed only when all other treatments and exercise programs have failed or when there is a clear surgical indication.

Historically, the most commonly performed operation for back pain has been spinal fusion. The basics of this surgery involve getting the painful piece of the spine to stop moving (if it can't move, it can't hurt), with fusion done along the back (posterior) or front (anterior) of the spine, although sometimes both approaches are necessary. Spinal fixation is usually combined with a bone graft. Full recovery can take more than a year, and the results are generally good, with patients experiencing a significant lessening of pain.

Disk replacement is a newer technique that has been done for years in Europe and is gaining favor in the United States. The procedure involves accessing the spine from the front of the body, removing the injured disk, and replacing it with artificial components. Disk replacement

Ways to Prevent Back Pain

- Exercise regularly to strengthen the muscles that support your back.

- Don't slouch.

- Maintain an ideal body weight.

- Don't worry . . . be happy! Studies show that people who are unhappy at work or home tend to have more back problems and take longer to recover than persons who have a positive attitude.

- Always stretch before exercise or other strenuous physical activity.

- Make sure your work surface is at a comfortable height.

- Sit in a chair with good lower back support and proper position and height for the task. Keep your shoulders back, switching sitting positions often and periodically walking around to relieve tension. A pillow placed behind the small of your back can provide some lower back support. If you need to sit for prolonged periods, rest your feet on a stool to reduce pressure placed on your disks.

- Wear comfortable, low-heeled shoes.

- Sleep on your side to reduce any curve in your spine; while firmer surfaces are generally better, make sure your mattress supports your lower back well while you sleep.

- Quit smoking. Smoking decreases blood flow to the spine and speeds up degeneration; it will also slow healing in the event you are injured.

is most indicated for disk disease involving the lower two disks in the lumbar spine, because replacing the disk allows the diseased spine segment to maintain some flexibility, which is especially helpful in this area of the body. The procedure requires a shorter recovery time than fusion because the bone does not need time to solidify, and early results have been promising.

Nontraditional Treatments

Many patients consider the following options when their back pain does not respond to traditional therapy. Not all have been scientifically proven to provide relief, but you may want to ask your doctor whether any of these therapies might be useful for your lower back pain. For more on alternative therapies, consult Chapter 10.

ACUPUNCTURE. The practice of Eastern medicine called acupuncture, in which thin needles are inserted throughout the body, is thought to trigger the release of naturally occurring painkillers within the body. Clinical studies assessing the efficacy of acupuncture for back pain are currently under way.

CHIROPRACTIC CARE. Some people swear by spinal manipulation, but talk to your physician about the most appropriate care for your situation. Be especially careful of aggressive spinal manipulation if you are older and osteoporotic (under certain circumstances, it is possible to sustain a spinal fracture from this procedure).

INTERVENTIONAL THERAPY. Injections of local anesthetics, narcotics, or steroids into soft tissues, joints, or nerve roots can ease chronic pain. Drugs may be given by catheter directly into the spinal cord.

TRACTION. Traction uses weights to apply constant or intermittent force in the hope of slowly improving skeletal structure alignment.

TRANSCUTANEOUS ELECTRICAL NERVE STIMULATION (TENS). This therapy involves placing small electrodes on the skin near the pain site to generate nerve impulses that will hopefully impede incoming pain signals. TENS is also thought to increase the brain's production of endorphins (natural pain relievers) that block pain perception.

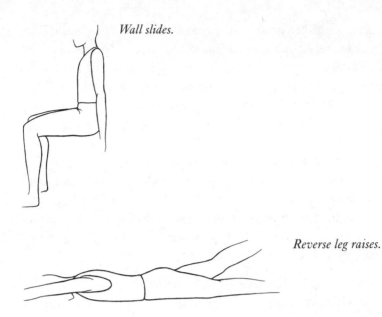

Wall slides.

Reverse leg raises.

ULTRASOUND. In this therapy, noninvasive ultrasound waves are passed through the skin in an effort to relax injured muscles.

Possible Future Therapies

A great deal of research is being performed to help doctors understand and treat low back pain. Some of the more exciting research involves new forms of "injectable" disk replacement as well as gene therapy research that may someday enable doctors to slow the spine's aging process.

Exercises for Prevention and Healing

There are several strengthening exercises that are believed to help avoid and treat lower back pain. Each of the exercises here is designed to be repeated five times.

WALL SLIDES. Stand with your back against a wall and your feet shoulder-width apart; slide down until your knees are just a few inches from the floor, bent to almost 90 degrees. Hold this position for five seconds, then slide back up the wall and relax.

REVERSE LEG RAISES. Lying on your stomach, tighten the muscles in one leg and raise it off the floor about a foot high. Hold this position for five seconds, lower the leg, and repeat with the opposite leg.

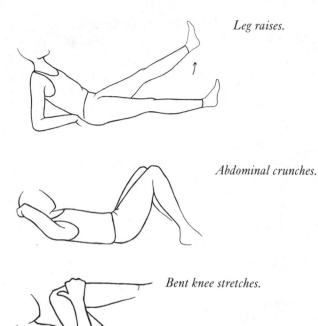

Leg raises.

Abdominal crunches.

Bent knee stretches.

LEG RAISES. Lie on your back with your arms at your sides and lift one leg off the floor about a foot high. Hold this position for five seconds before lowering the leg; repeat with your other leg.

ABDOMINAL CRUNCHES. Lie on your back with knees bent and feet flat on floor. Slowly raise your head and shoulders off the floor and reach both hands toward your knees, hold for five seconds, then lower your head and shoulders to the floor and relax.

POSTERIOR LEG SWING. Stand behind a chair with your hands on the back of the chair. Lift one leg back and up with your knee straight about a foot; return slowly to the floor. Repeat with the opposite leg.

BENT KNEE STRETCHES. Lie on your back and begin with your knees bent and feet flat on the floor. Raise your knees toward your chest, and place both hands under your knees. Slowly pull your knees as close to your chest as possible without raising your head. Lower your legs slowly, keeping your knees bent.

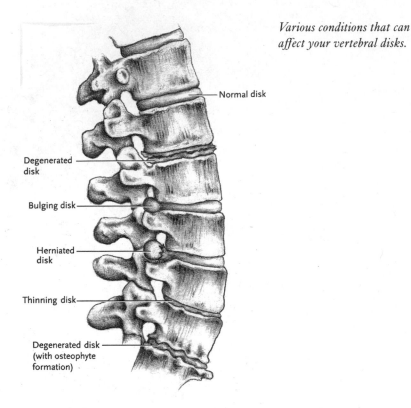

Various conditions that can affect your vertebral disks.

Normal disk

Degenerated disk

Bulging disk

Herniated disk

Thinning disk

Degenerated disk (with osteophyte formation)

HERNIATED DISK

A herniated disk (also known as a "slipped," or "ruptured," disk) is a common cause of neck, lower back, arm, or leg pain. Although a herniated disk can result from a single traumatic event, it is more often the result of a gradual degeneration of the spine.

Causes

As you age, your disks lose water and become more stiff and brittle. Sometimes the disks can also gradually swell and bulge out of the spine without losing fluid, a condition that does not necessarily cause pain. But when the tough outer covering of the disk tears, whatever the cause, the center of the disk may extrude, or herniate. And when the disk substance pokes out far enough to irritate a spinal nerve, you will almost certainly feel pain in your legs as well as in your back. This is called a slipped disk, although the disk actually remains attached firmly between the vertebrae and does not move.

Symptoms

Symptoms felt in the back include:

- Sciatica—a sharp, often shooting pain extending from the buttock down the back of one leg

- Weakness in one leg

- Tingling ("pins-and-needles") or numbness in one leg or buttock

- Loss of bladder or bowel control

- A burning pain centered in the back

Common symptoms felt in the neck include:

- Muscular pain between the neck and shoulder, possibly shooting down the arm

- Headache near the back of the head

- Arm weakness

- Arm tingling or numbness

- Loss of bladder or bowel control

- Burning pain in the shoulders, neck, or arm

Among the conditions that can weaken the disk are improper lifting techniques; obesity, which places extra stress on the disks; repetitive strenuous activities; smoking; trauma; and poor conditioning. In addition, you may have a genetic predisposition for herniated disks, which can make you more likely to experience a rupture.

The following symptoms require an urgent trip to your physician's office or an emergency room:

- Severe or worsening weakness of your muscles. For instance, if you were able to lift up your foot or stand on your toes after your injury but now you can't, injury to your nerve may be worsening and may require immediate surgery.

- Loss of bowel or bladder control. If you have lost the ability to control your urine, stool, or both (incontinence), there is too much pressure on the nerves that control your intestines or bladder, and surgery may be needed.

• Pain that is steadily worsening.

• Back pain with a fever.

• Pain that is worse at night or at rest.

Diagnosis

After obtaining a thorough medical history and carefully examining you, your doctor may order radiographic imaging of your spine. A traditional X-ray may pick up degenerative spine changes, but an MRI/CT scan or an EMG will be needed to determine whether there is any nerve damage.

Nonsurgical Treatments

Although pain from a herniated disk may feel like an emergency, most herniated disks do not result in permanent damage to your spine. Moreover, conservative therapy will relieve herniated disk symptoms in more than 90 percent of patients. This typically involves a regimen of bed rest and over-the-counter pain relievers; muscle relaxants, as well as analgesic and anti-inflammatory medications; cold compresses; and heat.

If conservative treatment fails, epidural injections of a cortisone-like drug may lessen nerve irritation and can be given on an outpatient basis.

Physical activity such as bending forward and lifting should be minimized; sitting for long periods should be avoided. The lower back exercises detailed earlier in the chapter may help strengthen your back and stomach muscles.

Surgical Treatments

Surgery is aimed at stopping the herniated disk from pressuring and irritating the spinal nerves; it should also relieve pain. But such remedies should be considered only if nonsurgical therapy does not lessen your symptoms after a period of at least six to twelve weeks, given the inherent risks of these invasive, open-surgery techniques:

LAMINOTOMY. In this procedure, only a portion of the lamina is removed to relieve pressure on a nerve or to allow the surgeon access to the disk that is pressing on a nerve.

LAMINECTOMY. The entire lamina is removed in a laminectomy, with your surgeon determining how much bone to remove by reviewing the MRI or CT scan.

DISKECTOMY. This technique involves removing part of a disk to relieve pressure on a nerve. In the case of a herniated disk, either a laminotomy or a laminectomy is usually performed along with a diskectomy.

MICRODISKECTOMY. Some surgeons are performing micro-diskectomies, which involve smaller incisions and the use of a microscope. The success rate for these operations is similar to standard diskectomy (80 to 90 percent), and the recovery time is somewhat shorter. Not all cases are suitable for this approach, however.

Alternative Therapies

Like sufferers of lower back pain, those patients who are searching for relief from pain resulting from a herniated disk often seek alternative treatments such as acupuncture, chiropractic care, interventional therapy, traction, TENS, and ultrasound. Be sure to consult with your doctor before beginning an alternative course of treatment.

Possible Future Treatments

Open diskectomy and microdiskectomy are the gold standards for surgically treating a herniated disk. But researchers are working on less invasive treatments, including:

NUCLEOPLASTY. With heat-producing (bipolar radiofrequency) technology, an energy field is created that lessens the pressure within the disk, providing pain relief.

OXYGEN-OZONE THERAPY. This therapy involves injecting a combination of oxygen and ozone gases into a herniated disk to reduce the disk's volume and limit pain. This treatment can enhance the effects of simultaneously administered steroid injections.

DISK AND NUCLEUS REPLACEMENT. Metal and plastic prostheses are being used experimentally as replacements for disks and nuclei.

BIOLOGICAL REPAIR. Although biological repair techniques are not yet considered safe enough for human use, there have been attempts to repair or regenerate a disk by injecting proteins that promote regeneration (for example, growth factor).

Note that because these procedures are still new (or in development), there are few long-term studies documenting their efficacy or safety. But it still may be worth asking your doctor whether any of these may be useful for your situation—either now or down the road.

Exercises for Prevention and Healing

Core strengthening builds the muscles that support your entire body. Pilates, yoga, and martial arts all provide well-rounded core strengthening programs. Other core strengthening exercises include:

TRANSVERSE CORE STRENGTHENING EXERCISE. This exercise strengthens the muscles that extend from your ribs across your waist and help support you in an upright position. Stand with your feet shoulder-width apart and toes turned in slightly while holding a ball directly in front of you. While keeping your abdominal muscles tight and your feet flat on the floor, turn your body from side to side. Repeat five to ten times; you may use progressively heavier balls.

SAGITTAL CORE STRENGTHENING. This exercise stretches and strengthens the low back muscles that help you stand and lift. With your feet shoulder-width apart and your arms by your side, stand about a foot from a wall, facing away from it. Tighten your abdominal muscles and, while keeping your hips and knees bent, lean back until your buttocks touch the wall. Using your hips, push your body back to an upright position, then extend your arms, reaching over your head. Repeat five to ten times.

ABDOMINAL CRUNCH. Inhale and draw in your stomach while lying on your back; exhale as you lift your chest off of the floor. Repeat ten to fifteen times.

Resistance training is exercise done against something that provides resistance, such as a weight (handheld weights or training machines) or isometric techniques (muscle-against-muscle resistance). The following exercises use resistance to strengthen the neck and back areas:

NECK PRESS. Press your palm against your forehead and use your neck muscles to push against your palm; hold for ten seconds and repeat ten times. Next, press your palm against one of your temples and use your neck muscles to push against your palm, holding for ten seconds and repeating ten times on each side. Finally, cup both

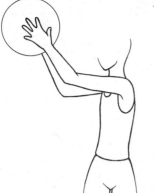

Transverse core strengthening exercise.

Neck press.

hands behind your head and use your neck muscles to press backward.

SIDE BRIDGE. While lying on your side, with knees bent at 90 degrees, prop your head up on your elbow, elongate your neck away from your shoulders, and draw in your stomach. Lift your hips away from the floor, keeping your head, shoulders, and hips in a straight line; hold this position for as long as thirty seconds (less if you feel too uncomfortable). Repeat five to ten times.

PRONE BRIDGE. Facing the floor, prop yourself up on your elbows and toes, keeping your shoulders, hips, and knees in a straight line. Hold this position for as long as thirty seconds. Repeat five to ten times.

COMPRESSION FRACTURES

When a compression fracture occurs, the normal height of the bones of the spine (vertebrae) is decreased.

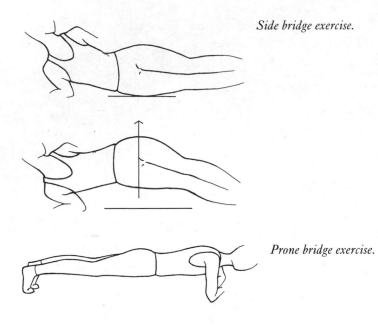

Side bridge exercise.

Prone bridge exercise.

Causes

Compression fracture injuries are most often due to osteoporosis, with the vertebrae collapsing within themselves and becoming flattened. These fractures most commonly occur in the mid- to lower back. But such injuries can also happen after a traumatic fall onto the feet that places an excessive load on one or more vertebrae. And, somewhat oddly, they sometimes occur for no apparent reason whatsoever.

Symptoms

Common symptoms of compression fractures are:

> Sudden pain at the time of fracture, ranging from mild to severe (sometimes there is no pain);
>
> Pain that worsens with prolonged sitting, standing, bending forward, twisting, carrying heavy objects, and walking;
>
> Pain that is brought on by sneezing and coughing;
>
> A hunchback-like curving of the spine (kyphosis), when multiple compression fractures occur;
>
> Rarely, damage to the spinal cord or nerves may produce weakness, numbness, paralysis, and loss of bowel or bladder function.

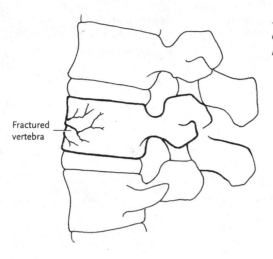

In a compression fracture, the osteoporotic vertebral body loses height.

Fractured vertebra

Diagnosis

A doctor can usually diagnose a compression fracture by taking a medical history and examining the back, although X-rays are generally used for confirmation.

Treatments

Pain relievers such as aspirin and nonsteroidal anti-inflammatory drugs can help, although opioids such as morphine are sometimes needed. If the fracture involves the lower back, wearing a brace may make walking less painful. Although patients may gravitate toward bed rest, walking as soon as possible can help speed recovery.

Although most compression fractures will heal on their own, an outpatient procedure to stabilize the vertebrae (called vertebroplasty) is sometimes used. After a local anesthetic is injected near the fractured vertebra, another needle is used to inject cement into the vertebra. The cement hardens in about two hours and stabilizes the vertebra, usually relieving pain. Kyphoplasty is a similar procedure that uses a balloon to expand the compressed vertebra before the cement is injected. Scientists and doctors are still assessing the safety and long-term efficacy of these treatments.

THE STINGER

A stinger (or "burner") is an injury to the nerves around the neck or shoulder; it is called a stinger because it produces painful electrical sensations

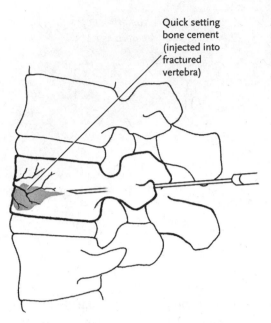

Quick setting
bone cement
(injected into
fractured
vertebra)

*In vertebroplasty, the fractured
vertebral body is stabilized with
injectable bone cement.*

in the arm. Although the stinger is an injury to the spine that commonly results from contact such as that which occurs in contact sports, it does not result in the paralysis seen in many serious spinal cord injuries.

Causes

The stinger injury occurs in one of two ways: one of the nerves connected to the spinal cord in the neck is compressed as the head is forced back and toward that side (think football and wrestling); or, the nerves in the neck and shoulder are overstretched as the head is forced away from the shoulder.

Symptoms

The stinger injury will produce sudden and severe painful stinging sensations in the affected arm; the pain usually lasts between seconds and minutes, although it can last for a few days. There is often associated weakness of the shoulder and arm muscles controlled by the injured nerve. A stinger tends to resolve promptly without intervention, but it can recur and, if not properly diagnosed and treated, can lead to persistent pain or even arm weakness.

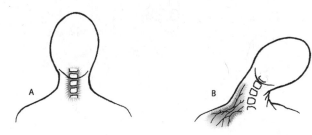

A stinger usually involves a temporary stretch injury to the nerves that control your arm.

Diagnosis

A doctor will ask detailed questions about the nature of the injury as well as perform a physical exam that includes an assessment of arm and shoulder strength. An EMG can sometimes be used to confirm muscle weakness and denervation, while an MRI may be ordered to rule out other causes of arm and shoulder pain.

Treatments

Treatment for acute pain from a stinger usually involves rest, ice or heat, pain medications, anti-inflammatory drugs, and, rarely, a cervical collar.

General Tips for Prevention

Many athletes who sustain a stinger exhibit abnormal postures that may delay recovery; these include jutting the head too far forward or rounding the shoulder too much. Learning to avoid these postures may speed recovery; in addition, physical therapy and massage can improve weakness and tightness.

BACK PAIN AND THE YOUNG ATHLETE

Although not common, back and neck injuries can occur in young athletes. Because the causes of back pain are different and potentially more worrisome in this population, we'll describe some of these more common back ailments here.

Muscular Strains and Ligament Sprains

Strains of the muscles and ligaments are the most common injuries that cause back pain in the young athlete. They can be caused by overuse, improper body mechanics and technique, lack of proper conditioning, insufficient stretching, and/or trauma. As the pain diminishes after the injury,

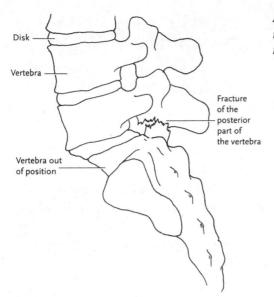

Disk

Vertebra

Fracture
of the
posterior
part of
the vertebra

Vertebra out
of position

*Spondylolysis can develop
when stress fractures occur in
the posterior spine.*

the athlete should be given exercises to assist in recovery, as well as to improve flexibility and strength so that similar injuries will be less likely. (During treatment, it is also important to maintain aerobic conditioning.) Before being released to return to active play, sport-specific exercises that mimic activities of the athletic competition are often included in the exercise program. It is also always important at that stage to evaluate and correct poor techniques that may have predisposed the athlete to the initial injury.

Spondylolysis and Spondylolisthesis

A stress fracture in a part of the vertebra called the pars interarticularis (spondylolysis) and the slippage of one vertebra in relation to another (spondylolisthesis) are common causes of back pain in the young athlete. While not seen exclusively in athletes, they are much more commonly seen in association with sports that require twisting and hyperextension of the spine (such as gymnastics). Pain is usually worse with arching of the back; consequently, the conditions can easily be mistaken for a simple strain or sprain. Because traditional X-rays are usually negative, a bone scan, MRI, or CT scan may be required to make the correct diagnosis.

Recovery usually involves rest, pain medication, and exercise; bracing may sometimes be required as well. Athletes with spondylolisthesis who have less than 50 percent forward slippage can usually return to all sporting activities after the pain resolves; athletes with more slip-page are strongly encouraged to change sports. Athletes with spondylo-listhesis should be monitored every six months for progressive slippage, particularly if they are still growing.

Disk Injury

Disk injury is much less common among young athletes, and back pain they experience may or may not be associated with sciatica. A careful his-tory and examination can diagnose a disk injury, while an MRI can de-finitively rule out other potentially serious causes of pain in this group of patients. Treatment of disk herniation in young athletes is similar to that of adults; most respond well to conservative therapy, and few will need surgery.

MAIN POINTS TO REMEMBER

- Most of us will experience some sort of back problem in our life-time.

- Healthy habits, such as exercising regularly, avoiding activities that add stress to the back, and maintaining proper body weight can go a long way toward avoiding painful back conditions as we age.

- A lot of new treatments are being developed for joint pain in the back, but not all have been proven beneficial. Be sure to consult your doctor before trying any alternative therapy.

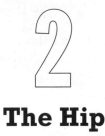

The Hip

THE HIP IS A ball-and-socket joint, linking the "ball" at the head of the thigh bone (femur) with the cup-shaped "socket" (called acetabulum) in the pelvic bone. The muscles and ligaments that circumvent and support the joint are considered part of it as well. Injuries to the hip can cause both acute and long-lasting joint pain. If you have an accident involving your hip or the muscles and ligaments that support it, it is essential that you give this important weight-bearing joint the care it needs. Here we explain the most common strategies for addressing joint pain in the hip, options that have improved in recent years with advances in both surgical and noninvasive approaches.

GROIN STRAIN

A groin strain is a partial tear of the small fibers of the adductor muscles, a group of three muscles that are considered part of the supporting cast of the hip joint: they start in the groin area and run down the inner thigh to the inner aspect of the knee. Thousands of professional athletes have been bothered by groin strains in their careers—a few examples include professional football players Terrell Owens and Randy Moss, and professional baseball player Barry Larkin—yet these injuries occur most com-

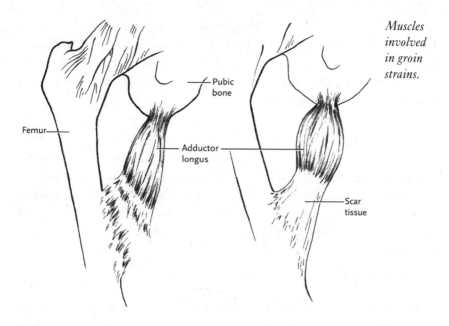

Muscles involved in groin strains.

Femur

Pubic bone

Adductor longus

Scar tissue

monly among poorly conditioned, poorly trained individuals who over-exert themselves on the playing field.

Causes

A groin strain can be caused by stretching the adductor muscles too much or too suddenly, overuse of the adductor muscles (think ice skaters), or a direct hit to the adductor muscles. Risk factors for a groin strain include:

Participation in sports that require bursts of speed like track and field, basketball, soccer, speed skating, and baseball;

Fatigue (many of us have played an extra game of volleyball or three-on-three basketball that we lived to regret);

Tight groin muscles, poor flexibility;

Cold weather.

Symptoms

Common symptoms of a groin strain are acute pain, tenderness, and stiffness in the groin area; weakness of the adductor muscles; and bruising (if blood vessels are broken), usually two to three days after the injury. (The bruising will often continue down the leg for several days, as gravity forces the swelling downward, but is nothing to be alarmed about.)

Diagnosis

A doctor will ask about your symptoms and how the injury happened. He or she will also examine your thigh for tenderness or bruising over the adductor muscles, and check you for pain or weakness when using those muscles, and for a limp when you walk.

Muscle strains are graded from 1 to 3 according to their severity, with Grade 1 tears being mild (just a stretch) and Grade 3 being the most severe (a complete tear). For severe groin strains, you may need an MRI to evaluate the extent of your injury, although it is not always necessary. Professional athletes often have MRI scans to help predict their time of recovery, but their situation is somewhat unique: when someone is paid millions of dollars to play a sport, a few hundred dollars for an MRI seems like small change.

Treatments

Although treatment will depend on the severity of the strain, it is typically divided into early and late components. Treatment during the first four days usually includes:

REST. Avoid activities that will cause pain, such as running, jumping, and weightlifting. Shorten your stride if walking hurts, and avoid playing sports until you are free of pain. Crutches may help rest your leg.

COLD. Apply ice or a cold pack to the groin area (fifteen minutes on and fifteen minutes off).

PAIN MEDICATIONS. Aspirin, ibuprofen (Advil, Motrin), or acetaminophen (Tylenol) can help relieve pain. Ask your doctor if you have any questions about using these medications.

COMPRESSION. Wear an elastic compression bandage (for example, an Ace bandage) high up on your thigh to prevent more swelling.

ELEVATION. Keep your leg elevated above your heart as much as possible for the first two to three days.

STRETCHING. When the initial pain decreases, start gentle stretching exercises as recommended by your doctor or physical therapist. Try to stretch several times a day.

By the fifth day, your doctor's recommended treatment is likely to include:

HEAT. Use heat before stretching to "warm up" your muscles.

STRENGTHENING. Strengthening is the last phase in recovery and should not be attempted until your doctor has determined that full flexibility has been restored. Returning too soon to strengthening can worsen your injury and delay your recovery.

General Tips for Prevention

If you've suffered a groin strain once, your risk of another episode of this very painful condition is unfortunately somewhat high. Prevention is therefore critical. And if you're lucky enough never to have had a groin strain, the following measures may help prevent you from getting one:

Keep your adductor muscles strong so they absorb the energy of sudden physical stress.

Incorporate specific adductor strengthening exercises into your workout routine.

Stretch your adductor muscles after a short warm-up period.

Learn the proper techniques for all of your exercise and sporting activities. This will decrease stress on all of your muscles, including your adductor muscles.

Exercises for Prevention and Healing

These exercises can be used to both treat the injured side and prevent injury to the uninjured side.

HIP STRENGTHENING EXERCISES WITH RESISTANCE. Tie one end of some elastic tubing around the ankle of your injured leg, and knot and secure the other end behind the base of a closed door. Facing away from the door, bring your leg forward about a foot, tightening your thigh muscles while keeping your knee straight. This exercise is called hip flexion. Next, while still attached to the elastic tubing, turn and face the door and pull your injured leg straight backward about a foot. This second exercise is called hip extension. Do three to five sets of both exercises, ten repetitions each.

HIP ADDUCTOR STRETCHES. While lying on your back with your knees bent and feet flat on the floor, slowly spread your knees apart. Make sure you are feeling your inner thigh being stretched, and hold this position for thirty seconds. Do five sets of ten stretches.

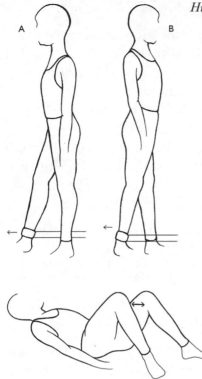

Hip strengthening exercise.

Hip adductor stretches.

HAMSTRING STRETCH. Raise your hurt leg up against a wall while lying on your back (if you do this while lying across an open doorway, your other leg can lie flat). Hold your hurt leg up against the wall at as close to a 90-degree angle as possible for about a minute. Repeat three to five times while feeling the stretch in the back of your thigh. This is a particularly difficult exercise and should be done gradually.

LEG RAISES. Lie on your injured side and bend your good leg over your injured one so that your foot will be flat on the floor and in front of your injured leg. Keeping your injured leg straight and the muscles of your thigh tight, lift the hurt leg about a foot off the floor and hold for five to ten seconds. Next, lie on your good side and again lift your hurt leg about a foot off the floor while keeping your thigh muscles tight. Do three to five sets of ten repetitions on each side.

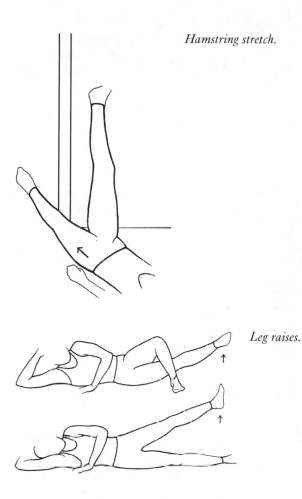

Hamstring stretch.

Leg raises.

HAMSTRING STRAIN

The hamstrings are a group of muscles (semimembranosus, semitendinosus, and biceps femoris) on the back of the upper leg that support the hip joint. Hamstring injuries are a common source of injury and chronic pain in athletes; just about anyone who has watched track events has seen athletes walking off the field clutching the backs of their thighs. Professional baseball stars Ken Griffey, Jr., Roger Clemens, and Mike Piazza have also all struggled with injuries to the hamstring muscles.

Hamstring injuries can be disabling, recurrent, and chronic; prevention is therefore the best treatment. As with groin strains, the severity of injury to the hamstring muscles is classified according to grades, with Grade 1 injuries being the least severe and Grade 3 injuries representing complete tears.

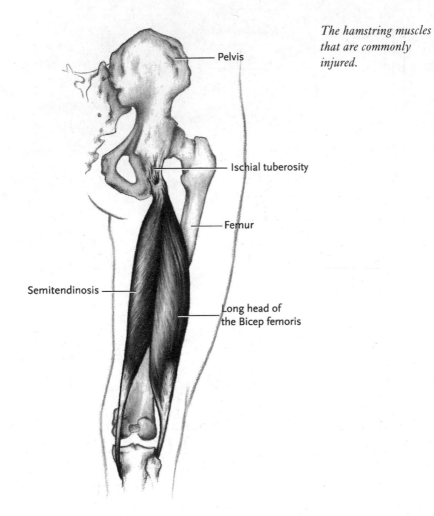

The hamstring muscles that are commonly injured.

Pelvis

Ischial tuberosity

Femur

Semitendinosis

Long head of the Bicep femoris

Causes

The major predisposing factors for hamstring strains are lack of warm-up, poor flexibility, and muscle fatigue. In addition, poor running style, especially overstriding, increases the risk of hamstring injuries in some runners. And perhaps surprisingly, the rapid growth that occurs during adolescence can lead to a tightening of the muscles that flex the hip and tilt the hip forward, which can increase the chances of developing hamstring injuries. For this reason, children in particular must stretch adequately and should not be overworked in practice or games.

Most hamstring injuries occur when these muscles are stretched eccentrically at high speed—that is, when a muscle is contracting yet being lengthened at the same time. One example of an eccentric contraction is the downward movement of a dumbbell in a bicep curl. Track-and-field events such as sprinting, as well as running in contact sports like football (which can result in direct blows to the hamstring muscle), are the typical culprits of hamstring injuries, which account for about a third of all lower extremity injuries in people between the ages of sixteen and twenty-five.

Symptoms

Hamstring injuries have distinctive symptoms:

> A sudden onset of pain or weakness in the back of a thigh, perhaps during an explosive movement such as jumping off the starting blocks in a sprint;

> A popping sound or a tearing sensation at the time of injury;

> Pain in the back of the thigh near the beginning or end of a sport activity;

> A sense of apprehension due to a sense of poor leg control after the injury;

> Pain upon sitting, or while walking uphill or climbing stairs;

> Swelling and bruising (with more severe injuries);

> With complete tears, the muscle may contract (curl up) into a noticeable lump in the back of the leg.

Diagnosis

Your physician will diagnose your hamstring injury based on a physical examination and on your description of how the injury occurred, and whether you feel pain when flexing your hamstring against resistance. In most cases, imaging procedures are not necessary to make an accurate diagnosis.

Treatments

Initial treatment of an acute injury to the hamstring will involve:

> PHYSICAL THERAPY. Patients with minor strains may go straight to strengthening exercises, whereas those with complete tears will need extensive treatment first. For as long as one week after the injury, the goal of therapy is to decrease pain, inflammation, and

swelling. The typical staples of treatment are rest, ice, compression (sometimes with elastic thigh bandages), and elevation (you may hear these four recommendations referred to by the acronym "RICE"). Most patients may begin active range of motion exercises after a couple of days; individuals with more serious injuries benefit from keeping the knee straight and immobilized for up to five days.

MEDICATIONS. Nonsteroidal anti-inflammatory drugs (NSAIDs) are usually started right away, with a narcotic (such as vicodin) sometimes prescribed as well for those with serious injuries and extreme pain. Past treatment options for hamstring injuries have included steroid injections directly into the muscle, but because of evidence of delayed healing and muscle loss, this procedure is no longer recommended.

SURGERY. In general, surgery may be recommended when there is an associated bone injury. Unfortunately, surgery for hamstring injuries can be challenging and unsuccessful.

CONSULTATIONS. With severe hamstring injuries, consultation with a sports medicine specialist or orthopedic surgeon is recommended.

Treatment one to six weeks after an injury usually focuses on improving the muscle's range of motion as well as on restoring flexibility and strength. Moist heat can warm up the muscle tissues before passive static stretching begins; electrical stimulation can be used for added pain relief. Next, you will begin a carefully guided exercise program in which resistance is increased gradually while exercise speed is decreased. Before returning to play, sports-specific training will be used to maximize your recovery and minimize your chances for additional injury. In general, your doctor will allow you once again to engage in your sport when the strength of the injured hamstring has at least 90 percent of the strength of the normal hamstring and you have regained full range of motion. Your strength, flexibility, and endurance should also be assessed to minimize the chances of reinjuring the hamstring—a serious concern since reinjury rates are as high as 80 percent, perhaps because of areas of calcification and inflammation in the hamstring after injury. (In addition, scar tissue may press on the sciatic nerve and cause what is called the hamstring syndrome.)

General Tips for Prevention

Warming up properly and maintaining flexibility and strength are crucial for preventing hamstring injuries. As fatigue sets in, the risk of injury increases because a fatigued muscle absorbs energy less efficiently. The risk of further injury can be decreased with improved form and by flexing the knee during activities whenever possible.

Exercises for Prevention and Healing

These exercises are designed to increase the flexibility and strength of the hamstring muscle. Each should be done three to five times in sets of ten, or until pain or excessive fatigue is felt.

HAMSTRING STRETCH AGAINST A WALL. Lying on your back across an open doorway, place the heel of your hurt leg up against the doorframe (while your good leg remains flat on the floor). Hold your injured leg up high against the doorframe for at least a minute, making sure you feel the back of your thigh stretch. The key to these stretches is to be gentle and patient. Increased flexibility will develop with time.

STANDING HAMSTRING STRETCH. Put the heel of your hurt leg on an approximately one-foot-tall stool that you've placed in front of the leg. Lean forward and bend from the hip until you feel the back of your thigh stretch. Hold this position for sixty seconds.

PRONE KNEE BENDS. Lying flat on your stomach, bend your injured leg at the knee and touch your heel to your buttock, then straighten the leg.

STANDING CALF STRETCH. Stand facing a wall at arm's length and place your hands against the wall at the level of your chest. Place the foot of your hurt leg twelve to eighteen inches behind your good leg, and lean into the wall (your good leg will be bent at the knee). Hold this position for about a minute.

TROCHANTERIC BURSITIS

A bursa is a fluid-filled sac that acts as a cushion between tendons, bones, and skin. The trochanteric bursa is located on the upper, outer area of the thigh. There is a bump on the outer side of the upper part of the thigh

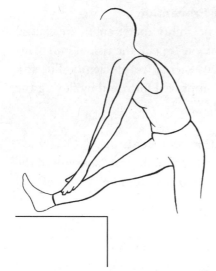

Standing hamstring stretch.

bone (femur) called the greater trochanter, over which the trochanteric bursa is located. Trochanteric bursitis is an irritation or inflammation of the trochanteric bursa.

Causes

The trochanteric bursa may be inflamed by a group of muscles or tendons rubbing over the bursa and causing friction against the thigh bone (femur). This injury can occur with running, walking, or bicycling, especially when the bicycle seat is too high. It can also be brought about by repetitive activities and overtraining.

Symptoms

When suffering from trochanteric bursitis, you have pain on the upper outer area of your thigh or in your hip. The pain is worse when you walk, bicycle, go up or down stairs, or lie on that side. Generally, you have pain when you move your thigh bone and are tender in the area over the greater trochanter.

Diagnosis

Your doctor will ask about your symptoms and examine your hip, back, and thigh.

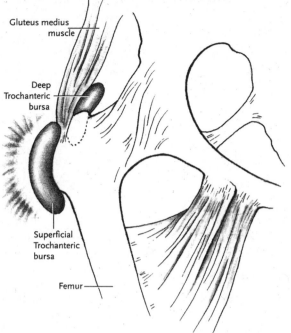

Gluteus medius
muscle

Deep
Trochanteric
bursa

Superficial
Trochanteric
bursa

Femur

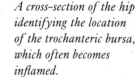

A cross-section of the hip identifying the location of the trochanteric bursa, which often becomes inflamed.

Treatments

Treatment may include rest or modification of activities or training; ice packs for twenty to thirty minutes every few hours for several days or until the pain goes away; anti-inflammatory medicine as prescribed by your physician; and/or a corticosteroid injection into the bursa to reduce pain and swelling.

While you are recovering from trochanteric bursitis, it is important to alter your routine to avoid exacerbating the injury. For example, you might try varying your exercise routine, perhaps by adding (or substituting) a low-impact activity like swimming.

The length of recovery depends on many factors, including your age, health, and history of previous injuries. Recovery time also depends on the severity of the injury; a bursa that is only mildly inflamed and has just started to hurt may improve within a few weeks, while a bursa that is very inflamed and extremely painful may take as long as a few months to heal. If you continue to perform activities that cause pain, your symptoms will return and you will take longer to recover.

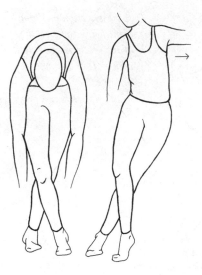

Iliotibial band stretch.

General Tips for Prevention

Trochanteric bursitis is best prevented by warming up properly and conditioning the muscles on the outer side of your upper thigh. Do not overdo your exercise; if you do, your body may force you to rest with a painful injury.

Exercises for Prevention and Healing

These stretching and strengthening exercises of the outer hip area will help keep your trochanteric bursa from becoming irritated. The stretches should be done three times each; the strengthening exercises are designed to be performed in three to five sets of ten.

ILIOTIBIAL BAND STRETCH (SIDE-LEANING). Stand sideways next to a wall, with your injured leg closest to the wall. Place the hand of your injured side on the wall for support, and cross your uninjured leg over the injured one, keeping the foot of the injured leg stable. Lean into the wall with your hip, hold the stretch for fifteen seconds, and release.

ILIOTIBIAL BAND STRETCH (STANDING). While standing, cross your uninjured leg in front of your injured one and bend down and touch your toes. If you can do so without pain, move your hands across the floor toward the uninjured side to feel more of a stretch on the hurt side. Hold this position for fifteen to thirty seconds and release.

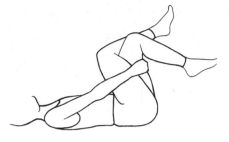

Piriformis stretch.

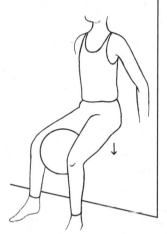

Wall squat with a ball.

PIRIFORMIS STRETCH. Lying on your back with both knees bent, rest the ankle of your injured leg over the knee of your uninjured one. Grab the thigh of your uninjured leg and pull that knee toward your chest; you will feel a stretch along the buttocks and possibly along the outside of your hip on the injured side. Hold this for fifteen to thirty seconds and release.

WALL SQUAT WITH A BALL. Stand with your back, shoulders, and head against a wall and look straight ahead. Keep your shoulders relaxed and your feet shoulder-width apart, one foot away from the wall. Hold a rolled-up pillow or a soccer-sized ball between your thighs. Keeping your head against the wall, slowly squat while squeezing the pillow or ball. Squat down until you are almost in a sitting position (your thighs should not quite be parallel to the floor); hold this position for ten seconds and then slowly slide back up the wall. Make sure you keep squeezing the pillow or ball throughout this exercise.

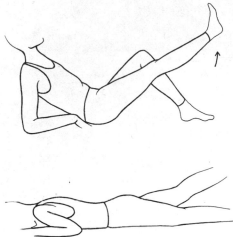

Straight leg raise.

Prone hip extension.

STRAIGHT LEG RAISE. Lie on your back, with your legs straight. Tighten the top of your thigh muscle on the injured leg and lift it about eight inches off the floor, keeping the thigh muscle tight throughout. Slowly lower your leg to the floor and relax.

PRONE HIP EXTENSION. Lie on your stomach with your legs straight. Tighten your buttocks and lift one leg off the floor about eight inches while keeping the knee straight. Hold for five seconds, then lower your leg to the floor and relax.

HIP FRACTURES

More than 350,000 Americans are hospitalized every year with a hip fracture—a serious and potentially life-threatening injury. In the past, half of those who suffered from a hip fracture died within a year of their injury due to direct and indirect medical and surgical complications. Today, with improved medical and surgical management, people can be back on their feet in a few weeks. Fortunately, surgery to repair a hip fracture is usually very effective, and even though recovery can be slow, many people, even those older than eighty, return to generally good hip health. The better your overall health and mobility, the better your chances for a complete recovery.

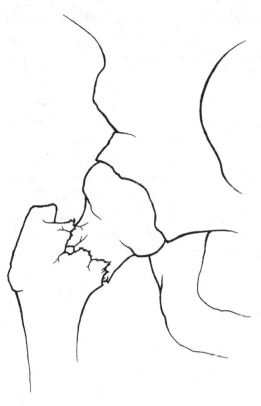

Typical fracture in an osteoporotic hip.

Causes

A combination of factors may increase your risk of a hip fracture, including:

AGE. The older you are, the more likely you are to suffer a hip fracture. As you age, your bone density decreases; your vision, hearing, and sense of balance worsen; and your reaction time slows due to diminished reflexes.

HEREDITY. Genetic factors influence bone size, bone mass, and bone density. A family history of osteoporosis or fractures later in life is a strong predictor of low bone mass. A small-boned, slender frame can put you at increased risk for osteoporosis; Caucasians (particularly Scandinavians) and Asians are much more at risk for osteoporosis than are African Americans.

SEX. Women are two to three times more likely than men to break a hip. This is because women lose bone density at a greater rate due to hormonal differences, their body build and constitution, and childbearing. In addition, menopause causes a dip in estrogen levels that promotes bone loss, increasing the risk of hip fractures as women get older.

CHRONIC MEDICAL CONDITIONS. Osteoporosis is one of the biggest risk factors for hip fracture. Loss of bone strength tends to be greatest in your spine, lower forearms, and upper thighbones (femurs)—the site of hip fractures. Medical conditions that can cause osteoporosis include hormonal problems (thyroid disorders); gastrointestinal disorders (including eating disorders, which may interfere with calcium and vitamin D absorption); rheumatoid disorders, which often lead to inactivity and loss of bone mass; and prolonged bed rest or immobility. In addition, chronic conditions that affect your nervous system, such as Parkinson's disease, multiple sclerosis, and seizure disorders, can increase your risk of falling and thus your chances of hip injury. People with decreased mental alertness (for example, those who suffer from dementia or depression) also have a greater chance of falling.

TOBACCO AND ALCOHOL USE. Smoking and alcohol abuse can interfere with the normal processes of bone building and remodeling, causing bone loss. These habits also interfere with the production of estrogen and testosterone, two hormones that work to increase bone mass.

NUTRITION. Lack of calcium and vitamin D in your diet when you are young lowers your peak bone mass and increases your risk of fracture later. In addition, women who are breastfeeding can experience a decrease in bone density; because of this, women should take calcium and vitamin D supplements during this time. Eating disorders such as anorexia and bulimia can damage your bones by depriving your body of essential nutrients needed for building bones.

MEDICATIONS. Long-term use of steroids may lead to an increased risk of osteoporosis. Thyroid medications and antiseizure medications can also promote bone loss or result in calcium or vitamin D deficiencies if used over a long period of time.

ENVIRONMENTAL HAZARDS. Check your house for cluttered floors, dim lighting, loose carpet or rugs, and dangerously placed electrical or telephone cords: these may increase your risk of stumbling and falling, which may in turn lead to an injury of the hip.

Symptoms

Signs and symptoms of a hip fracture include:

- Severe pain in your hip or groin
- An inability to put weight on your injured leg
- Stiffness, bruising, and swelling in and around your hip area
- A shorter leg on the side of your injured hip
- A turning inward of your leg on the side of your injured hip

Diagnosis

Your physician will ask for a history of the injury and will conduct a physical examination. X-rays are also used to make a conclusive diagnosis.

Treatments

Surgery is almost always the best way to repair a hip fracture. Nonsurgical alternatives are usually recommended only if you have another illness that would make surgery too risky. The type of surgery you will have generally depends on the part of the hip that is fractured, the severity of the fracture, and your age.

General Tips for Prevention

There are several ways that you can help yourself avoid the possibility of a hip fracture:

FIND OUT IF YOU HAVE OSTEOPOROSIS. If you have it, take steps to treat it. If you don't, work with your doctor (and follow the guidelines in this book) to try to prevent its occurrence.

DETERMINE YOUR CURRENT BONE DENSITY. If you find out early enough that your bone density is low, you can take steps to increase it and prevent complications such as a hip fracture down the road. We recommend a DEXA scan (short for dual energy X-ray absortiometry) for checking bone density. This painless procedure, conducted fully dressed, requires no premedication or advance dietary restrictions, and it administers less radiation than other scans—

even less than the amount of radiation that you would experience during a coast-to-coast airline flight. Ideally, these scans should be repeated every year or two. Ask your family doctor about the right time for you to have this screening performed.

MAKE GOOD LIFESTYLE CHOICES DURING YOUR YEARS OF PEAK BONE MASS. The higher your peak bone mass, the less likely you'll be to have fractures later in life. Maximum peak bone mass depends partly on genetics as well as on your exercise level and the amount of calcium you ingest. Bone mass peaks at about age thirty, after which you start to lose bone. Making the right life-style choices during peak bone-mass-building years and afterward will contribute to a higher peak bone mass and reduce your risk of osteoporosis later in life. In particular, be sure to take in enough calcium and vitamin D. Foods high in calcium include milk and other dairy products, dark green vegetables such as broccoli and spinach, citrus fruits, shrimp, and almonds. Vitamin D helps your body absorb calcium; this vitamin is made through your skin using energy from the sun. If you're considering calcium or vitamin D supplements, ask your doctor about an appropriate level for you. The recommended dietary allowance (RDA) for calcium for men and women over age fifty is 1,200 milligrams a day. The RDA for vitamin D for adults is ten micrograms daily until age seventy and fifteen micrograms daily after age seventy.

KEEP ACTIVE. Weight-bearing exercises increase bone density. Exercise also increases your overall balance and strength, making you less likely to fall.

DON'T DRINK EXCESSIVELY AND DON'T SMOKE.

WOMEN SHOULD CONSIDER HORMONE REPLACEMENT THERAPY (HRT). HRT slows the loss of calcium from your bones after meno-pause. Unfortunately, taking HRT can result in certain serious side effects and health risks, so check with your doctor to see if the risks outweigh the benefits for you.

FALL-PROOF YOUR HOME. Consider installing grab bars in your bathroom, stair treads on steps, and handrails along stairways. As you get older, you may want to consider a ranch house over a multi- or split-level home.

Dogs and Falls

We often see patients in their sixties or seventies suffer from falls and injuries incurred while walking their dogs — especially when the dogs are big and excitable. Exercise caution when walking your pet; if your pet is stronger than you are, you may end up suffering an inadvertent injury such as a hip fracture.

AVOID STRENUOUS AND DANGEROUS ACTIVITIES. Don't stretch to reach high places. Use a stepladder or, better yet, ask for help. Avoid lifting heavy objects, climbing, and engaging in unusually vigorous activities. We often see patients in the emergency room who have fallen while cleaning gutters or doing rooftop work that is best performed by a professional. While we can all understand the need to save a few dollars, the long-term cost of a serious injury can more than outweigh any short-term advantages. Refrain . . . to avoid long-term pain.

WEAR SENSIBLE SHOES. Older men and women should wear cushioned, flat-soled shoes with a flexible upper, such as sneakers. Avoid wearing high heels or sandals with light straps.

SEE YOUR EYE DOCTOR. Poor eyesight can contribute to falls, so have your eyes checked if you feel you may be having trouble with your vision.

BE MINDFUL OF MEDICATION SIDE EFFECTS. Weakness or dizziness, both of which are side effects of many common medicines, can increase your risk of falling. Talk to your doctor about the potential side effects of your medications.

WEAR A HIP PROTECTOR. These padded, externally worn protectors are similar to what hockey players wear to avoid injury. A study in the *New England Journal of Medicine* reported that wearing hip protectors reduced the risk of hip fracture from a fall by more than 60 percent; however, the protectors are cumbersome and may not be practical.

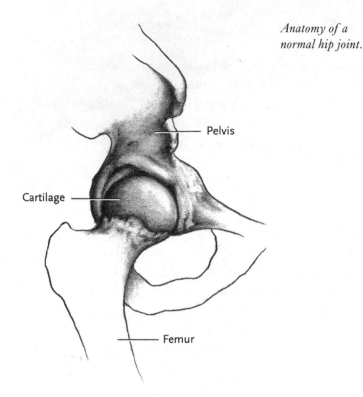

*Anatomy of a
normal hip joint.*

Pelvis

Cartilage

Femur

HIP ARTHRITIS

Osteoarthritis is the most common type of hip arthritis. As the protective cartilage in the hip is worn away, bare bone is exposed in the joint and causes pain and stiffness.

Causes

Hip arthritis usually afflicts patients over age fifty and is more common in patients who are overweight. Hip arthritis tends to run in families; trauma to the hip and fractures of the bones around the hip can also increase the risk of developing hip arthritis.

Symptoms

The most common symptoms of hip arthritis are pain, especially with moving the joint; stiffness; and walking with a limp.

Diagnosis

A doctor will begin an evaluation of a patient with hip arthritis with a physical examination and X-rays. A baseline X-ray can be compared with later exams to help monitor progression of the arthritis.

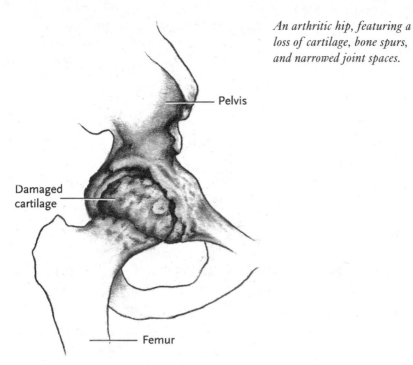

An arthritic hip, featuring a loss of cartilage, bone spurs, and narrowed joint spaces.

Pelvis

Damaged cartilage

Femur

Possible Nonsurgical Treatment Options for Hip Arthritis

Not all treatments for hip arthritis are appropriate for every patient. You should work closely with your doctor to determine which treatments are best for you. After this careful consultation, you may be advised to:

LOSE WEIGHT. While weight loss is probably the most effective therapy for hip arthritis, it is probably the least performed. Most doctors do not feel comfortable telling their patients that they are morbidly obese; in addition, most patients view surgical replacement as a quicker fix than weight loss.

MODIFY YOUR ACTIVITIES. Limiting certain activities or learning new exercise techniques may be helpful. Aquatic exercise is an excellent option for patients who have difficulty exercising because it strains the joints much less than exercise undertaken on land.

USE A WALKING AID. Using a cane or a single crutch in the hand opposite the affected hip can help reduce the demand placed on your arthritic hip.

DO PHYSICAL THERAPY EXERCISES. Strengthening the muscles around the hip joint may help decrease the burden on the hip; along

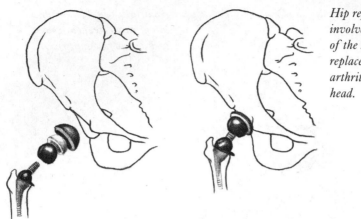

Hip replacement involves resurfacing of the socket and replacement of the arthritis femoral head.

the same lines, preventing weakness or atrophy of the muscles is an important way to maintain functional use of the hip. Unfortunately, physical therapy can sometimes make your symptoms worse.

TAKE ANTI-INFLAMMATORY MEDICATIONS (such as ibuprofen or aspirin).

CONSIDER SUPPLEMENTS. Glucosamine and chondroitin sulfate appear to be safe and may be effective for treatment of osteoarthritis, but research into these supplements has been limited.

Total Hip Replacement Surgery

During the surgical procedure called total hip replacement, the cartilage and damaged area of the hip bone are removed and an artificial implant—a hip prosthesis—made of metal alloys, ceramic, or plastic, is inserted to replace those injured parts.

The total hip prosthesis consists of three components:

1. A cup. Usually made of plastic, but sometimes of ceramic or metal, the cup replaces the similarly shaped hip socket.

2. A ball. The ball piece, which is always made of metal or ceramic, takes the place of the top of the femur.

3. A stem. Constructed of metal and inserted into the shaft of the bone, the stem adds stability to the prosthesis.

Less commonly, and usually in the case of a hip fracture rather than arthritis of the hip, a patient may be eligible for hemi-arthroplasty surgery. In this "half" surgery, only the head of the femur is replaced.

Did You Know?
Former president George H. W. Bush, golfing legend
Jack Nicklaus, opera star Luciano Pavarotti, and actress
Elizabeth Taylor had their hips replaced.

Hip replacement surgery is usually performed using general or spinal anesthesia. The typically six- to eight-inch incision is often made over the buttocks to expose the hip joint, after which the head of the femur is cut out and removed. The hip socket is then cleaned out and a new socket implanted, after which the metal stem of the prosthesis is inserted into the femur. The parts of the prosthesis are then pressed or, less commonly, cemented into place. Pain after surgery is usually eased through the use of patient-controlled analgesia (PCA), intravenous analgesics, or epidural (via the spinal cord) analgesics during the first three days after surgery. Later on, oral analgesic medications usually provide adequate pain relief.

If the procedure is elective (planned in advance rather than in response to an injury), patients can donate their own blood several weeks prior to surgery to replace any blood lost during the procedure. Sometimes, too, so-called cell saver techniques allow the blood that is lost during surgery to be sterilized and reinfused into a patient after surgery.

Although there has been a movement toward using minimally invasive or two-incision techniques for hip replacement surgery, it is still too early to tell whether this approach will become standard.

Are You a Candidate for Hip Replacement Surgery?

Most hip joint replacements are performed in people over the age of fifty, although many younger patients have had their hips replaced as well. Reasons for replacing the hip joint include:

- Severe pain from arthritis in the hip

- Fractures of the "neck" of the femur (most common in elderly patients)

By contrast, hip replacement surgery is typically not recommended for:

- Very young patients

- Patients with an actively infected hip

- Patients with neurologic (or nerve-related) disease affecting the hip (for example, polio or a spinal cord injury)

- Severely mentally challenged patients

- Patients who are extremely obese

Before you can undergo a hip replacement procedure, a thorough pre-operative evaluation will determine whether you are an appropriate candidate. Your physician will assess your degree of pain and disability, the impact of your disability on your daily life, and your medical health (including your heart, lung, liver, and kidney functions). If you are advised by your doctor that you are eligible for a hip replacement procedure, be sure to get a second opinion about whether it is the best option for you. If both of your doctors agree that you could benefit from the procedure, research the backgrounds of possible surgeons before making a commitment. In addition to learning what techniques he or she will use, you will want to know exactly how many hip replacement operations the surgeon has performed. Some studies have shown that patients of surgeons who perform fewer than twenty hip replacements a year have worse outcomes than those who are operated on by more experienced surgeons.

The Risks of Surgery

There are several important risks inherent in hip replacement surgery:

- Blood clots in the legs (deep vein thromboses) can dislodge and, in a potentially life-threatening condition, move to the lungs (pulmonary embolus)

- Nerve injury

- Pneumonia

- Infection, which may mean that further surgery will be required or even that the prosthesis will need to be removed

- Prosthesis dislocation

- Difference in leg length

Expectations and Care After Surgery

The results of hip replacement surgery are usually excellent. The operation relieves pain and stiffness, and most patients (more than 80 percent) need no help walking. Unfortunately, the artificial joint will loosen over time (although some hips can last as long as twenty years), and further surgery to correct problems will likely be needed as the hip ages. It is also possible that the lining of the new cup will become worn, necessitating replacement even before the prosthesis loosens (this usually happens in younger patients).

Walking and moving soon after surgery is strongly recommended. On the first day after surgery, you should get out of bed to a chair for at least an hour to improve circulation; when in bed, you will be instructed to perform ankle exercises regularly (your therapist in the hospital should show you these) in order to prevent blood clots.

Most people remain in the hospital for two to five days after surgery, although some patients may need to stay at a rehabilitation unit or long-term care center until their mobility has improved and they are able to live independently. Whether you will be able to return home directly after your surgery will depend on your age, general health, and support network at home, and whether your living situation requires that you navigate stairs.

Many surgeons place their patients on blood thinners for approximately six weeks after surgery to help prevent blood clots. These may be taken in the form of pills (either coumadin or aspirin) or injections (regular or low-molecular-weight heparin). The use of crutches or a walker may be necessary for as long as three months, although most people are able to walk without an aid several weeks after surgery.

Special Precautions to Avoid Hip Dislocations After Surgery

Your new hip will not be as stable as your original joint. While you will now have more range of motion without pain, the extremes of motion can put your hip at risk of dislocation (especially in the early postoperative period). Your physical therapist should instruct you about movements to avoid during the first six months after surgery. Most likely, you will be advised to

> Avoid crossing your legs or ankles even when sitting, standing, or lying down;

> Keep your knees below the level of your hips when you sit, and avoid chairs that are too low. Try sitting on a pillow to keep your hips higher than your knees;

> When sitting, keep your feet at least six inches apart;

When getting up from a chair, slide toward the edge of the chair and then use your walker or crutches for support;

Try to avoid bending over at the waist whenever possible. A long-handled shoehorn or a sock aid can help you put on and take off your shoes and socks without bending over. An extension "reacher" or "grabber" can also help pick up things too low for you to reach without bending over;

Place a pillow between your legs to keep the joint in proper alignment when lying in bed;

A special abductor pillow or splint may be used to keep the hip in correct alignment;

An elevated toilet seat can help keep the knees lower than the hips when sitting on the toilet.

MAIN POINTS TO REMEMBER

• When engaging in sports, be sure to warm up your leg and hip muscles thoroughly beforehand, and take a rest when you need it.

• Making good lifestyle choices during your peak bone mass years can help you avoid painful hip damage as an older adult.

• Be careful! Get help for strenuous jobs so that you won't risk injuring your hip, and set up your home so that you or your loved ones are unlikely to fall.

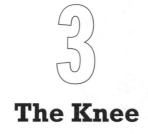

The Knee

KNEE INJURIES ARE EXTREMELY common among both the young and the old. According to the American Academy of Orthopaedic Surgeons, the number of physician visits in the United States for knee problems topped eighteen million annually, making knee injuries the second most common reason that people visit orthopedic surgeons (second only to spine or back problems). Understanding the anatomy of the knee, the activities that pose the greatest danger for that area of the body, and the most effective ways (immediate and long-term) to address damage to it will help you to prevent injuries as well as care for your knee in the event it requires medical treatment.

ACL SPRAINS

Ligaments are tough bands of fibrous tissue that connect two bones. The anterior cruciate ligament (ACL) and the posterior cruciate ligament (PCL) connect the thigh bone (femur) to the large bone of the lower leg (tibia) within the knee joint. The ACL and PCL form an "X" (hence the word "cruciate" in their names) inside the knee and stabilize it against front-to-back (anterior to posterior) or back-to-front (posterior to anterior) forces. An ACL injury consists of either a sprain or a tear and commonly occurs in people who participate in sports or skiing. The prognoses

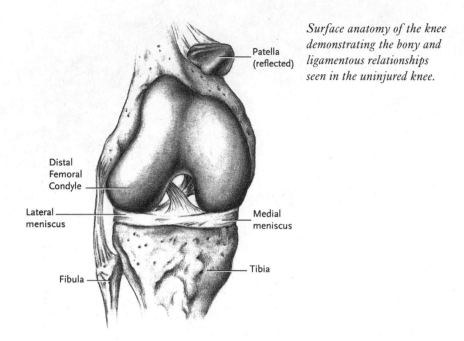

Surface anatomy of the knee demonstrating the bony and ligamentous relationships seen in the uninjured knee.

Patella (reflected)

Distal Femoral Condyle

Lateral meniscus

Medial meniscus

Fibula

Tibia

for these kinds of tears vary. You may remember that basketball standout Danny Manning was never the same after his ACL tear, whereas other athletes, like National Football League wide receiver Jerry Rice, do extremely well after undergoing surgery for their ACL injuries.

Like other types of sprains, ACL injuries are classified according to grades, with Grade 1 injuries representing partial tears and Grade 3 injuries describing complete tears. Unfortunately, most ACL injuries are classified as Grade 3, with only 10 to 25 percent being either Grade 1 or Grade 2. Currently, between 100,000 and 250,000 ACL injuries occur each year in the United States, affecting more than one in every three thousand Americans. Most of these injuries are related to athletic activities, and can be devastating to the athlete who may not be able to return to his or her previous level of play. (Fortunately, most weekend warriors can return, gradually, to their old form.)

Causes

In most cases, the ACL is torn by:

A sudden stop, twist, or change in direction at the knee joint. These movements usually occur during football, basketball, soccer, rugby, or skiing.

Extreme hyperextension (overstraightening) of the knee, which commonly occurs during awkward landings in basketball.

Direct contact. The ACL may be injured directly during contact sports (common examples include a sideways football tackle or a sliding tackle in soccer).

A motor vehicle accident. In these cases ACL injuries tend to be accompanied by much more significant knee injuries such as dislocations. Additionally, with coexisting dislocations or injuries that involve multiple ligaments, injury to the nerves or blood vessels is more common.

For reasons that are currently not well understood, women who play sports are seven times more likely than men to injure the ACL. Some have theorized that because women's hips are wider, the thigh bone (femur) comes down to the knee at more of an angle, placing additional stress on the ACL. In addition, estrogen is thought to make ligaments looser. One small study found a higher rate of ACL tears during the middle of a woman's menstrual cycle, when estrogen levels are at their highest. Compounding these potential problems, women generally have looser ligaments, which may increase the risk of ACL injury.

Symptoms

Symptoms of an ACL injury can include:

- Feeling a pop inside your knee

- Severe knee pain

- Significant knee swelling and tightness

- A black and blue discoloration around the knee from bleeding within it

- A feeling that your injured knee will "give out" if you try to stand or pivot

Diagnosis

Your doctor will ask you what movement caused the injury, how long it took for your knee to swell, and whether you felt a pop at the time of your injury. He or she will then examine both of your knees, checking your injured knee for swelling, deformity, tenderness, fluid inside the knee joint, and bruising. If your pain is not too great, your doctor may also check your knee's range of motion and strength. In the event your ACL ligament is torn, your injured lower leg will move much farther forward than your uninjured leg relative to your thigh bone and create the appearance of a protruding "lower lip" of the knee. The more your lower leg can be pushed forward from its normal position, the greater the amount of ACL damage and the more unstable your knee.

If your doctor thinks that you have an ACL injury, he or she will likely order a magnetic resonance imaging (MRI) scan of your knee joint to further evaluate the knee and the surrounding cartilage.

Treatments

To help patients remember all the components, the following set of techniques has often been referred to as the "RICE" treatment—rest, ice, compression, and elevation. It is used for many types of knee injuries and involves four steps:

- Rest the knee

- Ice the knee to reduce swelling

- Compress the knee with an elastic bandage

- Elevate the knee to decrease swelling

Your doctor may suggest that you wear a custom knee brace or take medications such as ibuprofen (such as Advil or Motrin) to relieve pain and swelling. Once your knee pain improves, you can start a rehabilitation program to strengthen the muscles around your knee and prevent stiffness. Surgery is often recommended and is necessary for younger patients who are athletic and want to return to sports that involve pivoting and jumping. Fortunately, surgery can be done on an elective rather than urgent basis.

While Grade 3 injuries are also initially treated with the usual rest, ice, compression, and elevation, as well as bracing and rehabilitation, the torn ACL must be reconstructed with either a piece of your own tissue (autograft) or donor tissue (allograft) once the swelling goes down (Grade 1 and Grade 2 injuries can be repaired by using tissue already within the knee). In the case of an autograft, the surgeon replaces your torn ACL with a piece of your own patellar tendon (tendon below the kneecap) or a section of tendon taken from your hamstring muscle. Today most knee reconstructions are done using minimally invasive arthroscopic (camera-guided) surgery, which uses smaller incisions and causes less scarring than does traditional open surgery.

ACL reconstruction is not a minor procedure. The risks of nerve injury, infection, bleeding, and reaction to anesthesia are still present. Reconstruction with a patellar tendon autograft also carries a small risk of anterior knee pain and possible fracture of the patella. After surgery there is the potential for developing stiffness, pain, and recurrent instability. Thankfully, the risks associated with ACL repair remain low, and most patients experience good to excellent outcomes.

General Tips for Prevention

Avoiding damage to the ACL will help ensure that you can enjoy participating in sports and ordinary daily activities without knee pain. Here are several techniques you can try at home to help strengthen and train your knee to prevent such injuries.

> Practice proprioceptive training. Proprioception is the ability to locate one's arms and legs in space without looking. Although it may be surprising, loss of proprioception is an extremely common cause of reinjury following knee and ankle trauma. It can also be a factor in initial accidents involving the ACL. The first significant study to show a reduction in ACL injury rates with proprioceptive training surveyed six hundred Italian male semiprofessional soccer players and found that even short periods of balance training during the four-to-six-week preseason period reduced ACL injury rates by over 700 percent. If you are interested in learning more about proprioceptive training, ask your doctor or physical therapist for guidance;

> Strengthen hamstrings by jump training and/or leg curls (after receiving your doctor's approval);

> Avoid turning and landing with straight legs;

> Warm up and stretch before participating in sports or exercising;

> Cool down and stretch after exercise;

> Increase your intensity gradually while training;

Heel slide.

Ask your sports-medicine doctor or athletic trainer about types of shoe cleats that may reduce your risk of knee injuries;

If you ski, use properly installed and adjusted two-mode release bindings (relatively standard on current skis).

Exercises for Prevention and Healing

The big leg muscles—the quads in the front of the thigh, and the hamstrings in the back—help stabilize the knee. Recent studies have shown that training programs that improve hamstring strength and knee stability markedly reduce the rate of ACL injuries. Each of the exercises that follow are designed to be done in three to five sets of ten. Please remember to consult with your doctor before beginning this or any other exercise regimen.

HEEL SLIDE. Sit with your legs straight in front of you and slowly slide the heel of your hurt leg toward your buttocks by pulling your knee to your chest, while keeping your heel on the floor. Release by slowly lowering your knee again.

PRONE KNEE FLEXION. Lie flat on your stomach. Slowly bend your hurt knee and touch your buttocks with your heel. Gently lower your foot to the floor to release. As you gain strength, you may find that you can add small weights to your ankle to further build your hamstrings.

HEEL RAISES. While standing, raise your heels off the floor and stand on the balls of your feet. Hold this position for three to five seconds before lowering yourself down. To strengthen your hamstring muscles even more, try standing on your injured leg alone.

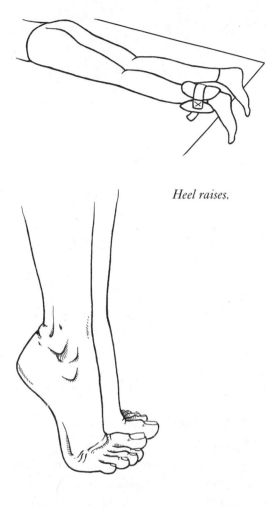

Prone knee flexion.

Heel raises.

WALL SQUATS. Stand with your back, shoulders, and head against a wall. Place a ball between your thighs and, while squeezing the ball, slide down the wall into a squatting position until your thighs are parallel to the floor. Hold for at least ten seconds and raise yourself back to a standing position.

HAMSTRING CURLS. Sit in a chair facing a door about three feet away, and tie one end of some elastic tubing around the ankle of your hurt leg. Knot the other end of the elastic tubing and secure it behind the base of a closed door. Bend your knee and slide your foot along the floor and under the chair, really stretching the rubber tubing before releasing.

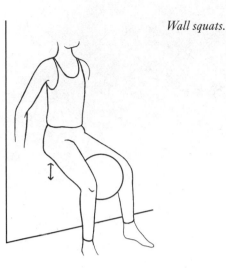

Wall squats.

MCL SPRAIN

The MCL is a strong band of tissue on the inner aspect of the knee that helps prevent sideways outward movement of the leg at the knee. It is often injured in football and skiing.

Like other ligament injuries, MCL sprains are classified according to grade, with Grade 1 sprains representing stretching of the ligament and Grade 3 sprains being complete tears.

Causes

Any motion that forcefully moves the leg outward at the knee can cause an MCL sprain. In addition, a hard blow to the outside part of the lower thigh can buckle a knee inward, injuring the MCL. Stiffness, poor conditioning, and overexertion can lead to MCL injuries. Moreover, trauma to the MCL is not always isolated. The anterior cruciate ligament (ACL) is injured in approximately 20 percent of Grade 1 MCL injuries and in as many as 80 percent of Grade 3 tears. The medial meniscus (the innermost knee cartilage) is injured 5 to 25 percent of the time (with the incidence increasing with the severity of the MCL injury); the patellar tendon is also injured in 10 to 20 percent of MCL injuries.

Symptoms

MCL injuries usually cause pain and mild swelling along the inner aspect of the knee; patients may feel that their knee is unstable. In addition, a person may feel a pop on the inner side of the knee during the injury.

Diagnosis

A physician will diagnose an MCL injury by asking questions about the injury and by conducting a thorough physical exam of the knee. In the event of a damaged MCL, the area will often be extremely tender when palpated by the physician. There will also be asymmetrical side-to-side motion in the knee, which should not occur in a healthy knee joint. If your doctor suspects an MCL injury after those initial screening tests, at least one X-ray will be performed to make sure there are no associated fractures; an MRI may also be done to assess the cartilage and other ligaments.

Treatments

Fortunately, most MCL injuries can be treated without surgery. The majority (even those that are Grade 3) are treated with rest, a brace, and physical therapy. The brace, which is typically worn for six weeks, is used to protect your knee against side-to-side stress on the MCL while walking. Rarely, and only for those cases that involve other ligament or cartilage injuries in the knee, surgery may be needed.

General Tips for Prevention

Keeping your leg muscles in tip-top shape may prevent some MCL sprains. Yet the braces some football players wear have *not* been shown to be effective. It seems that you cannot do very much to protect your MCL from a 250-pound person crashing into your knee.

Exercises for Prevention and Healing

Exercise may be somewhat helpful in speeding recovery from an MCL injury. In addition to the heel slide, prone-knee flexion, and wall slide moves that were described in the ACL section, you might try these additional movements to strengthen your damaged MCL:

> HIP ADDUCTION EXERCISES. These exercises involve adducting the hip—in other words, moving the hips closer together rather than farther apart. First, sit in a chair with your feet on the floor and your knees at a 90-degree angle—that is, with your thighs parallel to the floor and your lower legs extending straight down. Squeeze a pillow or ball between your knees for five to ten seconds before relaxing. Repeat ten to twenty times. Next, lie on the floor on your injured side, keeping your hurt leg straight. Bend your uninjured

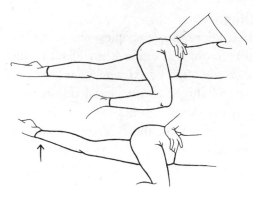

Hip adduction exercise.

Straight leg raises.

leg 90 degrees and place it over the injured leg, resting it on the floor. Raise your injured leg as high as possible and maintain this position for five to ten seconds. Repeat ten to twenty times.

STRAIGHT LEG RAISE. Lie on the floor with your hurt leg straight and with your other leg bent, foot flat on the floor. Raise your injured leg as high as possible while keeping your leg straight and your thigh muscles tight. Hold this position for five to ten seconds, and repeat ten to twenty times.

PCL SPRAIN

The posterior cruciate ligament, or PCL, prevents the lower leg (tibia) from slipping too far backward with respect to the thigh bone (femur), especially when the knee is bent. Most often the PCL is sprained because of a direct impact to the front of the knee, typically from a motor vehicle accident during which a knee hits the dashboard and is forced backward. During sports activities, the PCL can tear when an athlete falls forward and lands hard on a bent knee (which can occur in rugby, football, basketball, and soccer).

Interestingly, some degree of PCL damage occurs in as many as a third of all patients who are treated for knee injuries. Athletes seem to suffer PCL injuries most often, with football players and rugby players topping the list. Because a mild PCL sprain may not initially cause pain or movement problems in the injured knee, many athletes never seek medical care (the torn PCL may be discovered later, when tests are performed for an unrelated knee injury).

Symptoms

Symptoms of a PCL sprain include:

Considerable pain in the knee that does not go away within the first few hours after the injury;

Swelling of the knee that begins usually within twenty-four hours of the injury;

A feeling of looseness in the knee;

A feeling of unsteadiness and a tendency for the knee to give way, or an inability to bear weight on the injured leg;

A pop or the perception of something snapping or breaking at the time of the injury;

A feeling of fullness or tightness in the knee

Diagnosis

Your doctor will ask you to describe how you hurt your knee. He or she will want to know whether you had a recent serious impact to the front of your knee and, if so, the type of impact (for example, from a fall or an automobile collision), the position of your knee at the time of injury (flexed, extended, twisted), and the symptoms you are experiencing at that moment.

The doctor will examine both of your knees, comparing them as a way to better identify signs of swelling, deformity, tenderness, fluid inside the knee joint, and bruising. After assessing your knee's range of motion, the doctor will pull against the ligaments to check their strength. If your PCL ligament is torn, your lower leg will be able to be moved backward in relation to your thigh bone (femur). The more your lower leg can be displaced to behind its normal position, the greater the amount of PCL damage you have and the more unstable your knee.

If the results of your physical examination suggest that you have a PCL injury, you will need special diagnostic tests to further evaluate your knee. These may include standard knee X-rays to check whether the ligament has separated from bone, or an MRI to assess any soft tissue damage.

Treatments

Less serious PCL injuries are treated with physical therapy and bracing, while a complete PCL tear may require surgery if symptoms persist after therapy. Even so, many patients can live with a ruptured PCL without any noticeable disability. Like surgery for MCL and ACL injuries, PCL surgery reconstructs the ligament using either donated or the person's own tendons.

For all grades of PCL sprains, initial treatment involves rest, ice, compression, and elevation (RICE). Your doctor may also recommend a nonsteroidal anti-inflammatory drug (NSAID) such as ibuprofen (Advil, Motrin, or other brand) to relieve any mild pain or swelling.

After initial treatment with RICE, further treatment of PCL sprains depends on the grade of the injury. If you have a Grade 1 or a Grade 2 sprain, your knee may be splinted in a straight-leg position initially, after which you will begin an intense rehabilitation program to strengthen the muscles around the knee (especially the quadriceps) and support the knee joint. If the PCL is torn completely (Grade 3) and symptomatic, it can be reconstructed surgically using either a piece of your own tissue (autograft) or a piece of donor tissue (allograft). With an autograft, the surgeon typically replaces the torn PCL with a portion of your own patellar tendon (the tendon below the kneecap) or a section of tendon taken from the hamstrings. Almost all PCL reattachments and reconstructions are done using arthroscopic (camera-guided) knee surgery, which is less invasive than earlier techniques. After surgery to reconstruct the PCL, you will wear a long-leg knee brace and gradually begin a rehabilitation program to strengthen the leg muscles around the knee.

Overall, 50 to 80 percent of athletes with nonsurgically treated PCL injuries return to their sport at their preinjury activity level or higher after rehabilitation. Among patients who have surgical reconstruction of the PCL, more than 80 percent are able to return to their preinjury level of physical activity within three years of surgery. As a long-term complication, many patients with PCL injuries eventually develop pain from osteoarthritis in the injured knee joint. On average, arthritis symptoms begin fifteen to twenty-five years after the initial PCL injury.

General Tips for Prevention

To help prevent sports-related knee injures, you can:

- Warm up and stretch before you participate in athletic activities.

- Perform exercises to strengthen the leg muscles around your knee.

- Avoid sudden increases in the intensity of your training program. Never push yourself too hard, and increase your intensity gradually.

- Wear shoes that are appropriate for your sport.

PATELLAR TENDONITIS (JUMPER'S KNEE)

Patellar tendonitis, also called jumper's knee, is an inflammation of the patellar tendon (the tendon that extends over the kneecap and straightens the leg via the quadriceps muscle).

Causes

Patellar tendonitis is a strain of the patellar tendon, and it is most commonly caused by excessive jumping. For this reason, it is classically seen in basketball players—professional basketball star Vince Carter, for example, has been plagued by patellar tendonitis throughout his career. Other repetitive activities such as running, walking, or bicycling may also lead to patellar tendonitis.

In addition, patellar tendonitis can occur in people who have problems with the way their hips, legs, knees, or feet are aligned. This alignment problem can be caused by having wide hips, being knock-kneed, or having feet with arches that collapse when walking or running (a condition called overpronation).

If the patellar tendon ruptures, or tears completely, during strenuous activity, it is a catastrophic injury. For collegiate or professional athletes, it is generally career-ending.

Symptoms

The classic symptoms of patellar tendonitis are

Pain and tenderness around the patellar tendon;

Swelling in your knee joint or just below the kneecap, where the patellar tendon attaches to the shinbone;

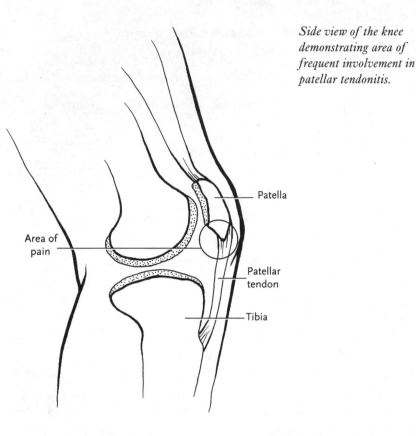

Side view of the knee demonstrating area of frequent involvement in patellar tendonitis.

Patella

Area of pain

Patellar tendon

Tibia

Pain when jumping, running, or walking, especially downhill or downstairs;

Pain when bending or straightening the leg.

Diagnosis

Your doctor will ask questions about your injury and examine your knee to see if you have tenderness at the patellar tendon. He or she will also have you do a straight leg raise as well as run, jump, or squat to see if any of these activities causes pain. To confirm the diagnosis, your physician may order X-rays or an MRI of your knee.

Treatments

Treatment for patellar tendonitis may include:

Applying ice to the knee for twenty to thirty minutes every three to four hours for two to three days or until the pain and swelling subside;

Immobilizing the knee;

Taking anti-inflammatory medication or a prescribed pain medication;

Wearing a band across the patellar tendon, called an infrapatellar strap, or a special knee brace to support your patellar tendon and prevent it from becoming overused or more painful. (You may have seen basketball players wearing these bands on their knees.);

Taping the knee;

Wearing custom-made arch supports (called orthotics) if overpronation is a problem;

Undergoing surgery, if the patellar tendon ruptures or does not respond to conservative treatment;

Cross-training—that is, varying your exercise routine to prevent overuse of the patellar tendon

General Tips for Prevention

Patellar tendonitis is usually caused by overuse during activities such as jumping or running or biking uphill, and is best prevented by having strong thigh muscles to absorb more of the shock of vigorous movement. In addition, you may want to avoid activities that aggravate the pattelofemoral joint, such as:

- Squatting
- Repetitive bending
- Sitting back on your heels
- Kneeling on your knee caps
- Excessive stair or hill climbing
- Wearing high-heeled shoes
- Riding a bicycle with a low seat
- Performing seated leg-extension exercises against resistance starting at a 90-degree knee bend

To help prevent injury to the patellar tendon, be sure to stretch before and after exercising, as well as vary your workout and sport activities.

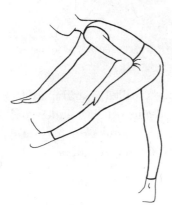

Standing hamstring stretch.

Exercises for Prevention and Healing

Doing exercises that strengthen the muscles around the knee can also be beneficial for preventing, and recovering from, patellar tendon injuries. Note that the hamstring stretch can be done at any time, whereas the quadriceps stretch should be performed only after the pain in your patellar tendon has eased. All of the exercises that follow are designed to be done in three sets of ten repetitions each.

STANDING HAMSTRING STRETCH. Stand and place the heel of your injured leg in front of you on a stool about fifteen inches high, keeping your knee straight. Lean forward, bending at the hips, until you feel a mild stretch in the back of your thigh. Hold the stretch for fifteen to thirty seconds.

QUADRICEPS STRETCH. Stand facing a wall at arm's length. Brace yourself by keeping the hand of the uninjured side against the wall. With your other hand, grasp the ankle of the injured leg and lift your heel gently toward your buttocks, keeping your knees together. Don't arch or twist your back. Hold this stretch for fifteen to thirty seconds.

SIDE-LYING LEG LIFT. Lying on your uninjured side, tighten the front thigh muscles of your injured leg and, keeping it straight, lift that leg eight to ten inches, then lower and relax.

QUADRICEPS ISOMETRICS. Sitting on the floor with your injured leg straight and with your other leg bent and the bottom of your foot on the floor, press the back of your injured knee into the floor

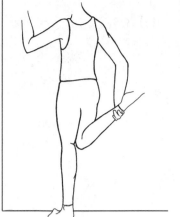

Quadriceps stretch.

Side-lying leg lift.

by tightening the muscles on the top of your thigh. Hold this position ten seconds, then release.

STRAIGHT LEG RAISE. Lie on your back with your legs straight. Tighten the top of your thigh muscle on the injured leg and lift that leg about eight inches off the floor, keeping the thigh muscle tight. Slowly lower your leg back down to the floor.

STEP-UP. Stand and place a support (like a block of wood), three to five inches high, under the foot of your injured leg while keeping your other foot flat on the floor. Shift your weight onto the injured leg and straighten the knee as you lift the uninjured leg off the floor. Slowly lower your uninjured leg to the floor.

WALL SQUAT WITH A BALL. Stand with your back, shoulders, and head against a wall, but with your feet one foot away from the wall and a shoulder's width apart. Place a rolled-up pillow or a soccer-sized ball between your thighs. Keeping your head against the wall, slowly squat while squeezing the pillow or ball until you are almost

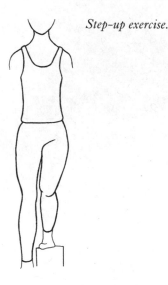

Step-up exercise.

in a sitting position (your thighs should not yet be parallel to the floor). Hold this position for ten seconds, then slowly slide back up the wall. Make sure you keep squeezing the pillow or ball throughout this exercise.

KNEE STABILIZATION. Loop a piece of elastic tubing around the ankle of your uninjured leg, and tie the ends together around a table leg or other fixed object. Facing the table, bend your injured knee slightly, keeping your thigh muscles tight. While maintaining this position, slide your uninjured leg straight back behind you, and then return it to its original position. Next, turn 90 degrees so your injured leg is closest to the table. Lift your uninjured leg slightly off the floor and move it away from your body, then return it to its original position. Turn 90 degrees again so your back is to the table. Lift and move your uninjured leg straight out in front of you, then return it to its original position. Finally, turn your body 90 degrees again so your uninjured leg is closest to the table. Lift and move your uninjured leg back and forth across your body.

RESISTED KNEE EXTENSION. Loop a piece of elastic tubing around the leg of a table or other fixed object and tie the ends together. Step into the loop and place the tubing around the back of your injured leg behind your knee. Lift your uninjured leg off the floor so that your injured leg is supporting your entire weight, and bend your injured leg at a 45-degree angle and slowly straighten, keep-

Knee stabilization exercises.

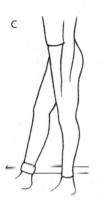

A

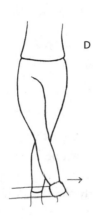

B

C

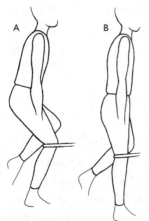

D

Resisted knee extension exercises.

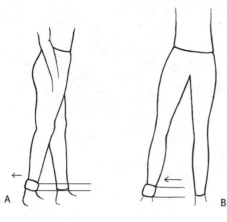

A   B

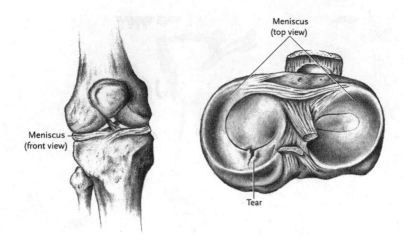

Normal and torn meniscus of the knee. The meniscus functions as a
stabilizer and shock absorber.

ing your thigh muscle tight. You can hold on to a chair for balance,
if necessary.

MENISCAL TEAR

The meniscus of the knee is a C-shaped piece of cartilage that curves
around the inner and outer aspects of the knee; it helps the knee joint
carry weight and also keeps your thigh bone (femur) from rubbing against
your shinbone (tibia).

Meniscal injuries are common. Moreover, because the cartilage of
the meniscus is poorly nourished by blood vessels (in fact, two-thirds of
the adult meniscus does not have a blood supply), meniscal injuries generally do not heal—and when the meniscus is injured, the weight of the
body is unevenly distributed throughout the knee joint, which can lead to
early arthritis of the knee.

Causes

Violent twisting, pivoting, cutting, and decelerating motions can lead to
meniscal injuries, particularly among athletes, and in this case often occur
in combination with other injuries such as torn ACLs. Meniscal tears can
also sometimes occur with the lifting of heavy objects, and, though rare,
older adults can tear their meniscus during repetitive movements such as
squatting.

Symptoms

A popping sensation may be experienced at the time of the tear. Most people can still walk on the injured knee, and many athletes can keep playing, but the injured knee will become painful and feel heavy and tight over the next twenty-four to forty-eight hours, as inflammation sets in.

Some patients may not even notice small meniscal tears, whereas others will experience a "locking" of the knee joint (if a flap of torn meniscus interferes with knee straightening). Other symptoms include knee pain, popping or clicking within the knee, swelling, tenderness when pressing on the meniscus, and decreased motion of the knee joint.

Diagnosis

If you think you have a meniscal tear, see your doctor for evaluation and treatment. Explain exactly what happened regarding the events leading up to your injury, and respond as thoroughly as possible to questions your doctor asks as he or she conducts a physical examination to evaluate your knee. Even if it seems likely that you have a meniscal tear, you will need to get an X-ray or MRI to rule out osteoarthritis or other possible causes of your knee pain.

Treatments

Treatment will depend on the size and location of the tear, and on how long you've had it. Your treatment may involve observation, the "RICE" techniques (rest, ice, compression, and elevation), anti-inflammatory medication, joint aspiration, or cortisone injection. In addition, surgery may be considered if less-invasive treatments are unsuccessful. In particular, arthroscopic treatment of a meniscal tear may be recommended if your symptoms do not improve or if your knee becomes increasingly painful, stiff, or locked.

In cases where surgery may be needed, your physician will determine—based on your injury, age, and other factors—whether to repair the meniscus or instead trim off damaged pieces of cartilage in a procedure called a meniscectomy. Meniscectomies are far more commonly performed than repairs because the surgery is a lot less complicated than a repair and because the meniscus heals so poorly (due to its poor blood supply). In addition, patients who undergo meniscectomy enjoy faster recovery times than those undergoing meniscal repair. The missing portion of meniscus, however, can lead to trouble years down the road. For this reason, arthroscopic repair, when successful, offers a better long-term prognosis than does meniscectomy.

A tear in the meniscus decreases the shock-absorbing capacity of the knee joint, increasing the risk of developing knee arthritis. After sustaining a meniscal tear, then, it is especially important to evaluate your lifestyle and activities, making any changes you can in order to prevent further injuries that could speed the development of arthritis in the knee. Maintaining good muscle tone through low-impact exercise, working to prevent trauma to the joint, and keeping a healthy, stable weight will all help to prevent additional damage to the meniscus.

PATELLOFEMORAL PAIN SYNDROME

People who have patellofemoral pain syndrome experience pain behind the patella, or kneecap, that is usually brought on with activity. The pain is typically most acute while walking downhill, descending steps, squatting, or sitting for long periods. People suffering from this syndrome sometimes report a popping sensation in their knees. One or both knees can be affected, and the syndrome is much more common in women and in people who are overweight.

Cause

The cause of patellofemoral pain syndrome is unknown but commonly attributed to a variety of factors, including overuse or overload, biomechanical problems, a misalignment of the hip or knee with the patella, and muscular dysfunction or weakness. In particular, the way your patella moves on the groove of your femur (known as the patellofemoral groove) is thought to play a role. Running or squatting exerts a force on the patella of seven to fifteen times one's body weight, so it is easy to see how such activities, when combined with underlying problems, can stress this area of the knee.

Diagnosis

Imaging (typically X-rays) may be considered in some cases to rule out conditions such as infection or malignancy and to confirm the diagnosis of patellar disease. In general, if there is no improvement after six weeks of committed therapy, particularly if the symptoms are in just one knee, X-rays should be considered.

Treatments

An initial conservative approach to patients with patellofemoral pain syndrome should include:

> Relative rest with possibly a temporary change to nonimpact or low-impact aerobic activity;

> Quadriceps and patella strengthening, and hamstring stretching, using the exercises described earlier in this chapter;

> Weight loss, if needed;

> An evaluation of footwear;

> Icing. Ice is the safest anti-inflammatory "medication," but its successful use requires discipline. If you are diagnosed with patellofemoral pain syndrome, you should apply ice for ten to twenty minutes after strenuous activity.

Note that some common remedies have not proven helpful for patellofemoral pain syndrome. These include taking NSAID medicines, taping the knee, and using knee sleeves and braces.

Surgery for patellofemoral pain syndrome is considered a last resort and usually involves a "lateral release," in which the amount of lateral pull on the patella is reduced; more complex surgery involves realignment of the patellar tendon.

KNEE ARTHRITIS

As the name implies, knee arthritis means arthritic symptoms in the knee joint. These may include pain in the tendons, ligaments, and pressure points between the bones.

Causes

Knee arthritis has a genetic component—that is, it runs in families—and typically affects patients over the age of fifty. It is also more common in patients who are overweight or who have had significant knee injuries.

Symptoms

The most common symptoms of knee arthritis are:

> Pain with activities;

> Decreased range of motion;

The Role of Obesity in Knee Osteoarthritis
While physicians have long suspected that being overweight
puts additional stress on the knees, recent studies have now
confirmed that obesity increases the risk for developing
knee osteoarthritis. Research conducted in 2004 by both
the Arthritis Foundation and the American College of
Rheumatology demonstrated that exercise and diet together
significantly improve physical function and reduce knee pain
in overweight people over the age of sixty.

Stiffness;

Swelling of the joint;

Tenderness along the joint;

A feeling that the joint may "give out";

Deformity of the joint (knock-knees or bowlegs). As arthritis progresses, the cartilage of the joint wears thin. The meniscus, or joint
cushions, are also damaged and wear away. If the damage is more
on one side of the joint than on the other, as is usually the case, the
knee will take on a deformed appearance. Moreover, when the knee
is worn more on one side, the forces transmitted across the joint are
altered: the healthier part of the knee is spared the burden of your
body weight, and the damaged portion carries the brunt of it. This
becomes a vicious cycle that leads to progression of the arthritis.
Note that when the inside, or medial side, of the joint is worn thin,
a varus deformity (bowlegs) will result. When the outside, or lateral side, of the joint wears thin, a valgus deformity (knock-knees)
develops. Women with the disease are more likely to have knock-
knees, whereas afflicted men usually have bowlegs.

Diagnosis

If you suspect you have knee arthritis, see your doctor for a thorough
physical examination and X-rays. These can serve as a baseline to evaluate
later examinations and determine if the disease is getting worse. An MRI
is not always necessary for diagnosis; particularly in cases of advanced

knee arthritis, the presence of significant symptoms may be enough to confirm the doctor's initial identification of the disease.

Nonsurgical Treatments

Treatment for knee arthritis ranges from gentle exercise to some of the most invasive knee surgeries performed, and may well include:

LOSING WEIGHT. It is important to realize that the less weight the joint has to carry, the less painful activities will be and the less articular cartilage damage will occur. Maintaining a healthy weight is one of the most helpful lifestyle commitments you can make for having healthy knees,

MODIFYING YOUR ACTIVITIES. Limiting certain activities may be necessary, and learning new exercise methods may be helpful. Water exercises are an excellent option for patients who have difficulty exercising;

USING A WALKING AID, SUCH AS A CANE.

UNDERTAKING PHYSICAL THERAPY. Strengthening the muscles around the knee joint may help decrease the burden on the knee, and preventing atrophy of the muscles is an important part of maintaining functional use of the knee. Physical therapy can be very painful for some patients, however, and should be avoided in these cases;

TAKING ANTI-INFLAMMATORY MEDICATIONS.

RECEIVING CORTISONE INJECTIONS. Injections of cortisone may help decrease inflammation and reduce pain within a joint. These can generally be given once every three months;

RECEIVING VISCOSUPPLEMENTATION. Injectable lubricants (such as synvisc and hyalgan) may be effective in treating the pain of knee arthritis and may even delay the need for knee replacement surgery (see Chapter 9);

TAKING NUTRITIONAL SUPPLEMENTS that may relieve joint pain in some people (for example, glucosamine and chondroitin sulfate).

Knee Replacement Surgeries

Exactly how effective arthroscopic surgery is for treating knee arthritis is uncertain. Although there are specific situations for which such an inter-

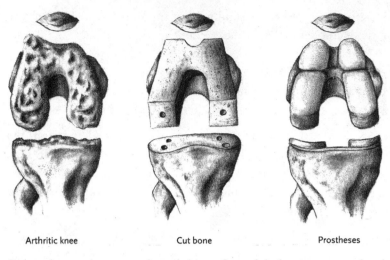

Arthritic knee   Cut bone   Prostheses

In most knee replacements, the arthritic surfaces of the knee are removed and the ends of the bone are capped with metal and plastic components.

vention may be useful, the appropriateness of surgery for knee arthritis has been an ongoing subject of debate.

In the total knee replacement procedure, the cartilage surrounding the knee is removed and replaced by a metal and plastic implant. The surgery is undertaken when symptoms are severe enough to warrant it.

Although there is no set age limit below which a patient cannot undergo full knee replacement surgery, if you are younger than sixty there is a high probability that the knee replacement will wear out in your lifetime, thus requiring revision knee replacement surgery. This is an important consideration because revision knee replacement surgery is generally not as successful as the first knee replacement, and rehabilitation from the second surgery is often more difficult.

When a complete knee replacement is performed, the bone and cartilage on the end of the thigh bone (femur) and on the top of the shinbone (tibia) are removed. Four pieces are then implanted: a femoral component, which fits on the end of the thigh bone; a tibial component, which fits on top of the shinbone (both the femoral and tibial components are usually made of cobalt-chrome metal, although some are made of ceramic); a plastic (usually polyethylene) component that fits between the femoral and tibial components; and a patellar component, made of plastic (also usually polyethylene) that replaces the cartilage under the kneecap.

Because knee replacement prostheses are made of metal and plastic, they will eventually wear out. Yet studies have consistently shown that knee replacement implants function well in 90 to 95 percent of patients even ten to fifteen years after surgery.

Full knee replacement surgery can be performed with general anesthesia, epidural (spinal) anesthesia, or a regional nerve block. The advantage of epidural and regional blocks are that pain medicine can be administered by these routes after the operation as well. Most patients use a PCA (patient-controlled analgesia) device to give themselves pain medicine intravenously for the first day or two following surgery.

Partial knee replacement surgery, also called a unicompartmental knee replacement, replaces only one part of the knee and is a valid surgical option for those with limited knee arthritis.

Risks of Knee Replacement Surgery

No surgery is without risk. The following are common but unwelcome side effects that may accompany knee replacement surgery:

> Blood clots in the large veins (deep venous thrombosis, or DVT) of the leg and pelvis are common after knee replacement surgery. To minimize the risk of developing blood clots, your doctor will start you on a blood thinning medication that will continue for several weeks after your surgery. In addition, you will be given compression stockings to keep the blood in the legs circulating. Early mobilization after the surgery will also help prevent blood clot formation.

> Infection following a knee replacement is a very serious complication that can occur either in the days and weeks following surgery (early infection), or even years down the road (late infection). An attempt to remove areas of infection surgically while leaving the implant in place is sometimes successful; however, some infections require removal of the implant followed by weeks of antibiotics given intravenously. Be sure to take any antibiotic medication given before, during, or after your surgery to avoid this dangerous complication.

> Stiffness. Because of scarring in the soft tissues around the knee joint, you may have difficulty bending your knee, sitting in a chair, or walking up and down stairs. It is therefore important to begin both bending and fully straightening the knee as soon as possible

after surgery, and to conscientiously follow a thorough physical therapy regimen for months afterward. If stiffness persists despite physical therapy, a manipulation under anesthesia may be performed to break up the scar tissue.

Implants can wear out and may loosen over time. Although new technology has considerably decreased this risk, loosening still occurs. Most knee replacements last an average of about twenty years, with some lasting less than ten years and some lasting more than thirty. Loosening is more of a problem in younger patients, who generally live longer and place more demands on the implanted joint.

General Tips for Prevention

Knee arthritis is best prevented by maintaining an ideal body weight, avoiding injuries, and conditioning your leg muscles to support the knee.

MAIN POINTS TO REMEMBER

- Knees bear an enormous amount of weight and stress

- Being overweight can contribute dramatically to the development of joint problems in the knee

- Those who experience a knee injury should seek medical help as soon as possible, both to take best advantage of the latest treatment options and to learn how to prevent reinjury

4

The Foot and Ankle

PEOPLE WALK ON AVERAGE ABOUT a thousand miles a year, and with each step they place up to 1.5 times their body weight on each foot. Vigorous exercise is even more demanding for the foot and ankle: in just one hour of strenuous exercise, our feet absorb up to one million pounds of cumulative pressure on no more than twenty-six bones. It is not surprising, then, that injuries to the foot and ankle are commonplace. In 2002, more than 12 million visits were made to a physician's office for foot, ankle, and toe problems; of these, 2.8 million were for ankle sprains and 1.2 million were for ankle fractures.

ANKLE SPRAINS

Sprained ankles are among the most common injuries in sports, with more than twenty-five thousand lateral ankle sprains occurring each day in the United States alone.

Causes

A sprained ankle can happen to anyone: athletes and nonathletes, children and adults. Ankle sprains account for a dramatic 15 to 20 percent of all sports injuries. Sports such as basketball, volleyball, soccer, gymnastics, and football have the highest incidence of this injury, with ankle

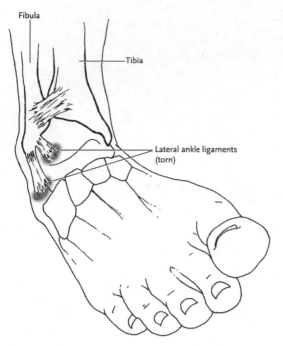

Fibula

Tibia

Lateral ankle ligaments
(torn)

*In an ankle sprain, the
ligaments on the outside
of the ankle are commonly
stretched and/or torn.*

sprains accounting for 25 to 50 percent of all injuries. Jumping, cutting, and pivoting place the foot at risk for turning inward (inversion trauma), causing a sprained ankle; close body contact between athletes also places the athlete's ankle at risk for inversion (for example, if a player steps on an opponent's foot).

The lateral (outer) ankle is more likely to be sprained, because the ligaments and bones in the inner ankle are much more stable than those of the outer ankle. This is why the foot is more likely to turn inward (ankle inversion) when you land on it awkwardly, causing a stretching or tearing of the lateral ankle ligaments.

Symptoms

Symptoms of ankle sprain include pain in the ankle, swelling and bruising, an inability to bear weight on the ankle, and, less commonly, numbness on the top of the foot.

Diagnosis

An X-ray may be required to determine whether you are suffering from a sprained ankle or an ankle fracture, but the diagnosis is usually made based solely on a doctor's examination and analysis of the circumstances of your injury. We recommend that you see a doctor even if you think you have only an ankle sprain, but you certainly should seek medical help if you are suffering from numbness in your toes or severe pain that does not improve over time, or if you are unable to place weight on your affected leg.

Nonsurgical Treatments

Ankle sprains, like all other ligament sprains, are graded from Grade 1 to Grade 3, with Grade 1 sprains being the mildest, and Grade 3 sprains the most severe.

For Grade 1 sprains, immediate treatment involves the "RICE" strategy (rest, ice, compression, and elevation):

Rest your ankle by not walking on it;

Ice should be immediately applied and used for twenty to thirty minutes three or four times daily;

Compression dressings, bandages, or Ace wraps should be used to immobilize and support the injured ankle and help minimize swelling;

The ankle should be elevated above the level of your heart for forty-eight hours. The less swelling you have, the less your ankle will throb.

For Grade 2 sprains, the same RICE guidelines apply, although more time for healing should be allowed. These sprains may require a physician's help; he or she may use a special device to splint or otherwise immobilize the injured ankle.

Grade 3 sprains can produce chronic instability, but surgery is rarely required. In addition to the RICE treatment, a short leg cast or a cast-brace may be used for two to three weeks. Rehabilitation is crucial in order to decrease ankle pain and swelling as well as to strengthen the ankle so that the injury will not recur. At first, rehabilitation exercises may involve active range of motion or controlled movements of the ankle joint without resistance; lower extremity exercises and endurance activities can be added as tolerated. Training in proprioception, the unconscious perception of movement and spatial orientation of the limbs—in other words, the ability to perceive the location of one's arms and legs in space without looking — is very important, because poor proprioception is a major cause of recurrent sprains and unstable ankles.

The treatment plan during the recovery phase, then, is aimed at regaining the full range of motion and strength in your ankle, as well as improved proprioceptive abilities. Strengthening begins with isometric (muscle against muscle) exercises and will advance to the use of elastic bands or surgical tubing. The goal is to improve strength in the four cardinal ankle motions: (1) dorsiflexion (turning your ankle upward so that your toes are pointing toward your head), (2) plantar flexion (turning your ankle downward, such as when you depress the gas pedal in a motor vehicle), (3) eversion (turning your ankle outward), and (4) inversion (turning your ankle inward). Strengthening of the peroneals (the tendons on the back and side of your ankle), which act as dynamic stabilizers of the ankle, is also vitally important. Nonsteroidal anti-inflammatory drugs (NSAIDs) can be used throughout the recovery process for relieving pain and reducing inflammation.

Surgical Treatments

Surgery for ankle sprains is rare and is used when injuries fail to respond to conservative therapy after months of rehabilitation. Using arthroscopy, in which a small camera is used to view the inside of the body, a surgeon will examine the ankle joint for loose fragments of bone or cartilage that were the result of trauma from ankle instability. If necessary, the surgeon will employ reconstructive techniques to repair any torn ligaments; this may involve the use of other ligaments and/or tendons (usually found in the foot and ankle area, although these can be from cadavers or from other parts of your body).

Unfortunately, studies have shown that at least 40 percent of acute ankle sprains cause some residual ankle symptoms six months after the injury. In addition, at least 10 to 20 percent of acute ankle sprains result in persistent ankle instability or pain.

General Tips for Prevention

The best way to prevent ankle sprains is to maintain good strength in the ankle, as well as overall muscle balance and flexibility. Balance and flexibility can be improved by adequately warming up before exercising, and by paying attention to walking, running, or working surfaces. A maintenance program of ankle strengthening, stretching, and proprioception exercises will help decrease the risk of future ankle sprains, particularly in individuals with a history of recurrent sprains or chronic instability.

Finally, wear appropriate shoes for your activity. The misuse of narrow cleats, which offer minimal arch support, or the use of running shoes for court sports, can increase your risk of ankle sprains.

Exercises for Prevention and Healing

As we mentioned earlier, maintaining good proprioception skills will help avoid falls—and sprains. Proprioception training begins with moving in a single plane and progresses to multiplanar exercises. In one of the earliest exercises, you will stand on your injured ankle with the foot and arch in a neutral position and hold your other foot off the ground. This exercise should be done near a wall to avoid falling.

Other useful exercises include the use of a balance, or tilt, board. While standing on the board you will attempt to balance your body while touching the board to the floor in a controlled patterns. Finally, you will move on to functional drills, jogging, sprinting, and cutting. The final step is figure-eight drills, which try to simulate sports-specific stresses on the ankle.

You may return to sports activities gradually, initially starting with in-line activities (for example, jogging) before progressing to forward-backward and side-to-side activities. Pivoting and "cutting" activities, which involve quick changes of direction for the ankle, should not be resumed until you are fully rehabilitated and comfortable with these activities.

HIGH ANKLE SPRAIN (SYNDESMOTIC LIGAMENT INJURY)

A high ankle sprain is an injury to the syndesmotic ligament—the broad ligament above the ankle joint that connects the tibia and fibula (the two bones of the lower leg).

Causes

The causes of high ankle sprains are similar to those of ankle sprains.

Symptoms

A high ankle sprain causes symptoms similar to other ankle sprains, but if you have this injury you will feel significant pain when your ankle is externally rotated (turned to the outside), or when your calf is squeezed.

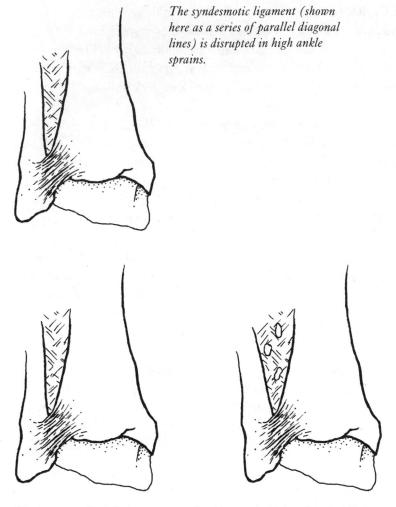

The syndesmotic ligament (shown here as a series of parallel diagonal lines) is disrupted in high ankle sprains.

The image on the left shows a normal ankle; on the right, there is a high ankle sprain. The space between the tibia (the large bone) and the fibula (the thinner bone), is widened in the sprained ankle.

Diagnosis

In addition to standard ankle X-rays, special stress views of the ankle should be done if this injury is suspected. These views will check for any abnormal widening between the tibia and fibula.

Treatments

High ankle injuries do not heal as well or as quickly as routine ankle sprains. These injuries need to be evaluated by an orthopedic surgeon to determine whether nonsurgical or surgical treatment is most appropriate. Nonsurgical treatment involves applying a non-weight-bearing cast for about six weeks, whereas surgery involves placing a screw through the skin between the tibia and fibula to hold the bones in the appropriate position while the ligament heals. After about three months, the screw may or may not be removed in a second operation (your surgeon should discuss with you the benefits and drawbacks of this option in your particular circumstance).

ANKLE FRACTURE

The ankle joint is made up of three bones: the tibia, fibula, and the talus. The tibia is the main bone of the lower leg and is the medial, or inside, ankle bone. The fibula is a smaller bone that parallels the tibia in the leg and is the lateral, or outside, ankle bone. And the ends of the tibia and fibula closest to your feet form a joint with the top of the talus (one of the bones in the foot).

While lateral ankle sprains are extremely common, ankle fractures are thankfully less so; they make up only 15 percent of all ankle injuries.

Causes

There are many ways you can fracture your ankle:

- Violently rolling or twisting the ankle inward or outward

- Flexing or extending your ankle joint in an extreme manner

- Landing straight down on your ankle with severe force

- Suffering direct trauma to the ankle

Symptoms

The following signs and symptoms indicate a possible ankle fracture and warrant immediate assessment in the emergency room:

- Gross ankle deformity

- Visible bone

- Intolerable or worsening pain

- Inability to move your toes

- Complete numbness of the foot

• Complete inability to move your ankle

• Cold or blue foot

As you might expect, pain is the most common complaint of ankle fracture, but if you have such a fracture you may feel the pain in your foot or leg rather than in the ankle itself. Although you can also have associated fractures of your foot (especially on the side of the small toe) or outer aspect of your knee when you fracture your ankle, it is typically ankle pain that will stop you from walking. Ankle swelling frequently occurs as well, and may suggest either soft tissue damage with blood around the joint, or fluid (such as blood) within the ankle joint itself. Bruising may or may not occur immediately, and will generally track down toward your toes or the soles of your feet. Deformity of the ankle is also a telltale sign of fracture. And although infrequent, nerve or blood vessel (neurovascular) injuries can occur with ankle fractures and may result in numbness, paleness, extreme pain, or the inability to move your foot or toes. The more violent the injury, the more likely you are to have associated neurovascular damage.

Diagnosis

Diagnosis of an ankle fracture is made by physical examination and by X-ray. Your doctor will perform a physical exam, looking for

Bruising, abrasions, or cuts;

Swelling, bleeding, or soft-tissue damage;

Pain, deformity, grinding of bones, or movement of broken bones within the knee, shin, ankle, or foot;

Fluid in the joint or joint instability;

An inability to feel a pulse in the ankle area or other evidence of injured vessels;

Impaired sensation and movement in your leg, ankle, or foot.

If a broken bone is suspected, ankle X-rays will be performed, and if additional fractures are a concern, your doctor may request X-rays of your knee, shin, or foot as well.

Treatments

Some minor ankle fractures do not require a splint or cast and are treated like a mild ankle sprain. More typically, however, treatment of ankle fractures involves either placing a splint or cast on your injured ankle or performing surgical repair. The type of repair needed and the length of time that you will need to immobilize your ankle depend on several factors, including age, health status, activity level, smoking history, bone quality, and severity of the injury. For example, if your bone has broken through your skin, your fracture is called a compound fracture. Because of an increased risk of infection, compound fractures are much more serious than simple ones and require intravenous antibiotics, operative debridement (removal of loose or traumatized tissues), and close subsequent monitoring by your surgeon. Most ankle fractures take six to twelve weeks for the bones to heal completely; it may be as long as a year before full use and range of motion within the joint are regained. More severe fractures, especially those requiring surgical repair, can take even longer to heal. Unfortunately, all fractures increase your likelihood of future development of arthritis in the affected joint.

Ankle rehabilitation with physical therapy should begin after your surgeon is confident that the joint can once again move safely. The exercises used and the rate of progress through rehabilitation will generally vary based on the fracture pattern, your age, the healing rate, and the ankle's stability. Patients are often asked to perform guided calf stretching and strengthening exercises, along with range-of-motion activities that emphasize regaining the four cardinal motions of the ankle (dorsiflexion, plantarflexion, inversion, and eversion).

ACHILLES TENDON RUPTURES

The gastrocnemius and soleus muscles are the two large calf muscles that generate the power to push off with your feet or to walk on tiptoe; the Achilles tendon connects these two muscles to your heel. Achilles tendon ruptures are tears in this important tendon in the back of the ankle.

Causes

Because the gastrocnemius and the soleus are used constantly while you are walking or running, it is not surprising that the Achilles tendon can occasionally become inflamed from overuse. Although the Achilles tendon is the strongest and largest tendon in the body, sports that tighten the calf muscles (such as basketball, running, and high-jumping) can overstress this tendon and cause a strain (Achilles tendonitis) or rupture. Direct trauma to the foot, ankle, or calf can also cause Achilles tendon in-

Did You Know?

• The Achilles tendon is named after the Greek god Achilles, who was vulnerable only at his heel.

• The Achilles tendon can withstand a force of a thousand pounds or more.

• Some scientists have theorized that our long Achilles tendon evolved as part of a group of features that long ago helped humans become better runners, and thus better at finding food.

juries. Players engaged in sports that involve repetitive jumping are at an increased risk for Achilles tendon ruptures; it makes sense, then, that approximately 75 percent of all Achilles tendon ruptures occur during sporting events such as basketball, baseball, or soccer.

Although Achilles tendon ruptures can occur in highly trained professional athletes, they more commonly occur in so-called weekend warriors. These part-timers are often in poor physical condition and tend to overstress their tendons recklessly. Poor footwear can also contribute to Achilles tendon stress and rupture; players should avoid footwear with insufficient heel height, rigid soles, inadequate shock absorption, or uneven wear. Sudden increases in training intensity, excessive training, and training on hard surfaces should also be avoided.

Achilles tendon ruptures most often occur when an individual pushes off his or her weight-bearing foot while extending the knee joint (as during sprinting or jumping). They also can happen when the ankle is abruptly dorsiflexed (when the foot points toward your head)—for example, if you accidentally step into a hole, fall forward, or descend rapidly from considerable height.

But these injuries do not always occur as a result of trauma; age and lack of use can cause the tendon to grow thin, weak, and susceptible to damage. People who have high cholesterol levels or diabetes, or who are taking certain medications such as steroids, are more susceptible to Achilles tendon ruptures.

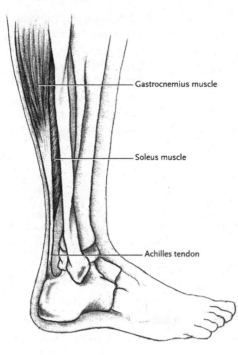

Gastrocnemius muscle

Soleus muscle

Achilles tendon

The Achilles tendon is the largest tendon in the body, and is a confluence of the gastrocnemius and soleus muscles.

Symptoms

There are several characteristic features of an Achilles tendon rupture, although not all of these have to be present for such an injury to have occurred:

- Sensation of a sudden snap in the back of the calf or heel
- Sudden, severe pain
- Bruising and weakness after the initial pain, swelling, and stiffness
- Swelling in the calf
- Inability to run, climb stairs, or stand on your toes
- Inability to press down with your foot (for example, to depress the gas pedal in a motor vehicle)
- A gap in the tendon that appears approximately an inch or two above the heel bone

Diagnosis

A physical examination by a doctor, who will also inquire about the history of the injury, is usually sufficient to make the diagnosis of an Achilles tendon rupture.

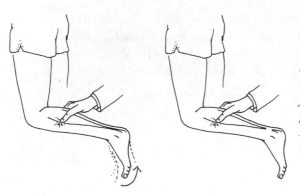

The Thompson test is used to diagnose Achilles tendon ruptures. When the calf is squeezed by the examiner, the foot should push away from the body in a normal patient. In patients with Achilles tendon ruptures, no motion occurs.

The classic finding is a palpable and painful defect about an inch or two from where the tendon connects to the heel bone along the back of the foot. Also, there is often bruising in the area of the tear and very weak plantar flexion (inability to stand on one's toes or to point the toes downward). Unfortunately, however, Achilles tendon rupture is often misdiagnosed as a strain or minor tendon injury because of swelling and because some still have the ability to point their toes. Other tendons in the leg may permit this pointing (although weakly), confusing even experienced practitioners.

A simple test can indicate whether the Achilles tendon is intact; when someone squeezes your calf muscles while you lie on your stomach, your foot should point down (because the tendon is still connected to your calf muscles). If there is still a question about whether the tendon is intact, ultrasound and MRI can help confirm the extent of the injury.

Nonsurgical Treatments

If surgery is not required, you will usually begin your recovery with a cast that will immobilize the Achilles tendon for six to eight weeks. The cast is then removed, and gentle range-of-motion exercises are initiated. Strengthening exercises are generally started over the following two weeks, with a resumption of sports by four to six months after the injury. It may take a year or longer to regain full strength in the tendon, and, unfortunately, some residual weakness is common.

The disadvantages of nonsurgical therapy include potential weakness due to prolonged immobilization, a loss of strength due to lengthening of the tendon, and reported rerupture rates of as high as 18 to 30 percent.

Surgical Treatments

Operative intervention is usually recommended for young, healthy, and active individuals. Most semiprofessional or professional sports athletes are strongly encouraged to undergo surgical repair of their Achilles tendon ruptures in order to minimize future rerupture rates—indeed, surgery offers a dramatic 96 to 99 percent chance of permanent recovery. In general, then, surgery is indicated in younger patients and high-functioning athletes, and in cases of large partial ruptures, acute ruptures, or recurrent ruptures.

General Tips for Prevention

Good conditioning and proper stretching can aid in the prevention of Achilles tendon injuries. You should properly warm up your Achilles tendon before participating in activities that place it at risk.

ACHILLES TENDONITIS

Achilles tendonitis involves inflammation, irritation, and/or swelling of the Achilles tendon.

Causes

Common causes of Achilles tendonitis include:

- Rapidly increasing your running distance or speed

- Participating in jumping sports like basketball

- Adding hill running or stair climbing to your training routine

- Inadequate overall conditioning (for example, restarting a full exercise routine too quickly after a lengthy break)

- Trauma caused by sudden and/or hard contraction of the calf muscles (such as when putting forth extra effort in a final sprint)

- Overuse resulting from the natural lack of flexibility in the calf muscles

Symptoms

Symptoms of Achilles tendonitis range from mild to severe and include:

- Mild pain after exercise or running that gradually worsens

- A feeling of sluggishness in your leg

- Episodes of diffuse or localized pain, sometimes severe, along the tendon while running (or a few hours afterward)

- Tenderness, usually most severe in the morning, about an inch or two above where the Achilles tendon attaches to the heel bone

- Stiffness that tends to improve as the tendon warms up with use

Diagnosis

Diagnosis of Achilles tendonitis will be made largely based on your description of the injury and on findings during the physical exam; in particular, your physician will look for tenderness along the tendon. Imaging studies are rarely needed, although MRI or ultrasound tests can help to assess the degree of tendon involvement and rule out other sources of pain such as arthritis.

Nonsurgical Treatments

The initial therapy for Achilles tendonitis usually involves nonsteroidal anti-inflammatory drugs (NSAIDs) and physical therapy to stretch the muscle-tendon unit and strengthen the muscles of the calf. Activities that aggravate symptoms will need to be limited.

Recovery is slow, and a cast or brace is sometimes used to immobilize the heel and allow the inflammation to decrease. But if you fail to take your treatment seriously and continue vigorous activity, you will risk a complete rupture of the tendon.

Surgical Treatments

If conservative treatment fails to improve your symptoms, surgery may be needed to remove inflamed tissue from around the tendon and to remove any irreparably diseased parts of the tendon. When necessary, surgery has been shown to be very effective in easing pain.

General Tips for Prevention

There are six ways you can help yourself avoid Achilles tendonitis:

Focus on stretching and strengthening your calf muscles;

Warm up gradually (perhaps by walking) before running or participating in other strenuous activities;

Choose your running shoes carefully;

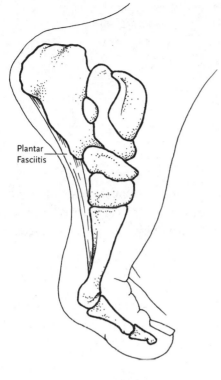

Plantar
Fasciitis

In plantar fasciitis, there is inflammation of the fascia on the bottom of the foot near the heel.

If you increase your running distance or speed, do so at a slow rate (no more than 10 percent a week is a good rule of thumb);

Begin new activities gradually;

Cool down properly after exercise.

PLANTAR FASCIITIS

Plantar fasciitis is a common, painful foot condition that occurs when the band of tissue that runs from the heel along the arch of the foot becomes inflamed. It generally affects middle-aged men and women and is often confused with heel spurs (when extra bone material forms on the heel bone). In reality, heel spurs are usually painless and are of unknown significance in the treatment of plantar fasciitis.

Causes

Plantar fasciitis occurs when the plantar fascia—the thick, ligamentous connective tissue that runs from the heel to the ball of the foot—becomes

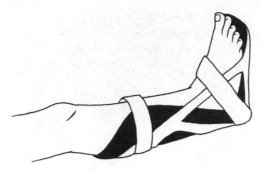

Night splint used to treat plantar fasciitis.

inflamed. This strong and tight tissue contributes to maintaining the arch of the foot; it is also one of the major transmitters of weight across the foot as you move. It is therefore not surprising that obesity and repetitive stress can damage it.

Symptoms

The pain from plantar fasciitis is most severe when you first stand on your feet in the morning, and, although the pain tends to diminish quickly, it usually returns after prolonged standing or walking.

Diagnosis

Plantar fasciitis is usually diagnosed based on physical examination and the information you provide about where and when the pain occurs. An X-ray is taken only if an associated injury is suspected.

Treatments

Surgery and steroid injections are rarely needed and usually not recommended for plantar fasciitis. Instead, more conservative approaches are usually relied on to provide relief. These approaches include:

- Rest
- Ice applied to the heel area for fifteen to twenty minutes at a time, as directed by your doctor
- Anti-inflammatory medications
- Shoe inserts

In addition to these familiar remedies, your doctor may recommend the use of night splints or the administration of extracorporeal shock wave therapy (ESWT). Night splints keep the back of the leg and heel ex-

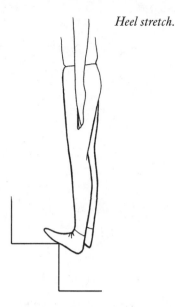

Heel stretch.

tended while you sleep, thereby decreasing arch contraction at night and (hopefully) pain in the morning. ESWT is a new treatment that uses energy pulses to induce microtrauma to the tissue of the plantar fascia. Much like the treatment used for breaking up kidney stones, it is thought to help in the body's tissue repair process. Although ESWT is not usually among the first therapies considered, it can be helpful in those cases where more traditional techniques have been tried and were unable to provide relief.

General Tips for Prevention

Custom orthotics can help if there is a structural problem with the foot, but adequate stretching and strengthening exercises are the most effective ways to prevent plantar fasciitis.

Exercises for Prevention and Healing

ARCH STRETCH. While lying on your back, loop a towel around the ball of your foot and stretch the arch with the heel of your foot on the ground. You should feel the plantar fascia stretching, but it should not be painful. Hold for ten seconds, release, and repeat three to five times for each foot.

STEP STRETCH. Stand on a step and let your heels hang over the edge. Holding on to a railing for balance, lower your heels and let

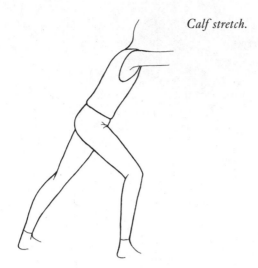

Calf stretch.

your calves and arches stretch. Hold this position for ten seconds, release, and repeat three to five times for each leg.

CALF STRETCH. Lean against a wall with your arms outstretched; hold your back knee straight, lean into the wall by bending your arms. Hold, release, and repeat.

TURF TOE

Turf toe is usually caused by either jamming the toe or pushing off repeatedly while running or jumping; pain at the base of the big toe is the result, although stiffness and swelling may also occur. The condition is so named because it is common among athletes who play sports on artificial turf (commonly football and soccer players).

Causes

In turf toe injuries, the capsule surrounding the joint at the base of the toe rips. This tear can lead to instability of the joint at the base of the toe, with eventual loss of cartilage and possibly the onset of arthritis.

Diagnosis

Your doctor can diagnose turf toe based on your account of the injury and on a physical examination. X-rays may be indicated to rule out a fracture or arthritis in the big toe.

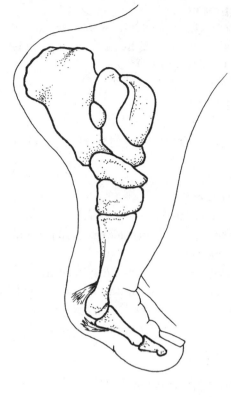

Turf toe involves a tearing of the capsule surrounding the base of the big toe.

Treatments

Treatment of turf toe involves resting the sore toe, icing the area, and elevating the foot; anti-inflammatory medications may be used for pain. Sports should be avoided for around three weeks to allow the joint capsule tear to heal; special inserts can be used to limit the motion of the big toe and to prevent further damage to the joint capsule once play is resumed. Even with this care, however, turf toe often recurs.

Hallux Rigidus

Hallux rigidus is the medical name for arthritis of the big toe. The joint at the base of the big toe is called the metatarsophalangeal (MTP) joint; it is the most commonly affected area of arthritis in the foot.

Causes

Arthritis of the big toe will sometimes follow an earlier traumatic injury (even years after the event), or it will be associated with a systemic condition like gout or osteoarthritis.

Symptoms

Characteristic signs of hallux rigidus include pain and/or swelling at the base of the big toe; pain when you raise up your big toe; or pain in the big toe that increases with activity, particularly with running or jumping.

Diagnosis

The mobility of your MTP joint will be compared to that in your opposite foot to see how much motion is lost; X-rays are taken to assess for severity of the arthritis.

Treatments

Generally, your doctor will first recommend that you take anti-inflammatory medications and wear shoes with firm soles that will prevent motion at the base of the big toe. If those treatments do not work, surgery may be recommended. The two most common surgical procedures for hallux rigidus are chilectomy (removal of the bone spurs that are impeding the motion of the joint) and arthrodesis (fusion). Fusion permanently immobilizes the joint and eliminates the arthritis pain; this measure is used when the arthritis is extensive.

General Tips for Prevention

If your big toe is injured, carefully follow any treatment advice to help yourself avoid arthritis later. Women may also want to avoid high-heeled shoes, which can exacerbate the condition.

FOOT AND ANKLE ARTHRITIS

There are over thirty joints in the foot, and if arthritis develops in one or more of them your balance and gait may be impaired. In addition to the metatarsophalangeal joint of the big toe (discussed earlier), the joints most commonly affected by arthritis in the foot and ankle are the ankle (tibiotalar joint), where the shinbone (tibia) rests on the uppermost bone of the foot (the talus); the three joints of the hind foot; and the midfoot (metatarsocunieform joint), where one of the forefoot bones (metatarsals) connects to the smaller midfoot bones (cunieforms).

Symptoms

The classic symptoms of foot and ankle arthritis are:

- Pain

- Stiffness or reduced motion

- Tenderness

- Swelling

- Difficulty walking

Diagnosis

A diagnosis of foot or ankle arthritis is made largely on the basis of a physical examination and on your description of your problem, although your physician may also perform a gait analysis. In addition, X-rays, CT, and MRI scans may be ordered to show changes in the spacing between bones or in the shape of the bones themselves.

Nonsurgical Treatments

Your doctor may recommend some of these nonsurgical treatments for foot or ankle arthritis:

- Pain relievers or nonsteroidal anti-inflammatory medications

- Appropriate shoe inserts

- Custom-made shoes, such as stiff-soled shoes with a rocker bottom

- An ankle-foot orthotic

- A cane

- Physical therapy

- Steroid injection into the joint

Surgical Treatments

Several surgical treatments are available to those suffering from arthritis in the foot and ankle.

Arthroscopic surgery may be somewhat helpful in the early stages of arthritis, when used for a process called arthroscopic debridement. Tiny probes and shavers are inserted through small incisions to clean the joint area by removing foreign tissue and bony outgrowths (spurs).

Noisy Joints
Joint cracking, common in the ankles and knees when
walking up steps, is usually a benign condition. While the
sound may cause you some alarm, you are not damaging your
joints when this noise occurs—that is, as long as no pain is
involved. Noise associated with pain should be evaluated by
a physician.

Arthrodesis, or fusion surgery, eliminates the joint completely by
fusing the bones together; because fusion eliminates motion, pain
should theoretically disappear as well. Surgeons will make use of
pins, plates, screws, and/or rods as well as grafted bone to help
secure the fused area.

Your orthopedist may recommend replacing the ankle joint with
artificial implants in cases of severe and refractory arthritis. Keep
in mind, however, that total joint replacement in the ankle is not
as advanced or as successful as total hip or knee joint replacement
(and is still not performed routinely at many centers). Likewise,
joint replacement for the big toe is not recommended at this time.

MAIN POINTS TO REMEMBER

• Ankles are weaker on the outside than on the inside.

• Sprained ankles are among the most common injuries in sports,
with more than twenty-five thousand lateral ankle sprains occurring each day in the United States alone.

• High ankle sprains do not heal as well or as quickly as do routine
ankle sprains.

• If you are going to participate in sports involving jumping, pivoting, or running, be sure to choose the right footwear for the activity.

• Although the Achilles tendon is the strongest and largest tendon
in the body, sports that tighten the calf muscles (such as basket-

ball, running, and high-jumping) can overstress this tendon and cause a strain (Achilles tendonitis) or rupture.

• Plantar fasciitis is a common, painful foot condition that occurs when the band of tissue that runs from the heel along the arch of the foot becomes inflamed. It generally affects middle-aged men and women and is often confused with heel spurs.

• Be careful to follow your doctor's advice regarding treatment of injuries to the foot, ankle, and toe in order to minimize the risks of later arthritis in those areas.

The Shoulder

THE MUSCLES AND TENDONS in your shoulder provide continuity between your upper arm bone (humerus) and your shoulder blade (scapula); they also help hold the ball of your upper arm bone in your shoulder socket, much like a golf ball rests on a tee. Yet the arrangement and flexibility of these muscles and tendons help allow your shoulder to have the greatest range of motion of any joint in your body. Perhaps this great freedom of movement explains why the shoulder seems to be so easily damaged. Common shoulder injuries include rotator cuff tears, soft tissue tears known as labral tears, "frozen shoulder," dislocated shoulder, and shoulder arthritis.

ROTATOR CUFF TEARS

Rotator cuff tears are a common cause of pain and disability in adults. The rotator cuff is made up of four muscles and their tendons that combine to form a "cuff" over the upper end of the arm (head of the humerus), and its function is to help lift and rotate the arm and to stabilize the head of the humerus within the shoulder joint. The four muscles in the rotator cuff — the supraspinatus, infraspinatus, subscapularis, and teres minor — originate from the scapula, and together they form a single tendon unit that

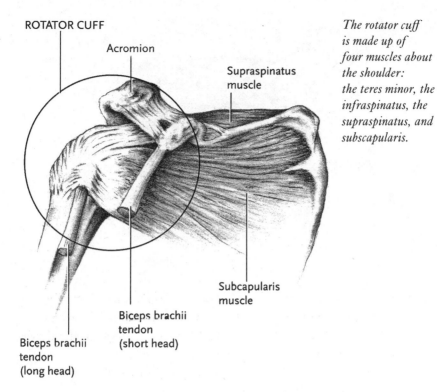

ROTATOR CUFF

Acromion

Supraspinatus muscle

Subcapularis muscle

Biceps brachii tendon (short head)

Biceps brachii tendon (long head)

The rotator cuff is made up of four muscles about the shoulder: the teres minor, the infraspinatus, the supraspinatus, and subscapularis.

works synchronously. Most rotator cuff tears occur in the supraspinatus muscle, but other parts of the tendon may be involved.

Causes

Rotator cuff injuries are fairly common in patients over age forty and usually occur due to falling, lifting, or repetitive overhead arm activities (such as reaching up to place something on a shelf, throwing a baseball, or working overhead). Younger patients may also suffer rotator cuff damage due to acute trauma or repetitive overhead activities, and sometimes a cuff tear may happen along with another injury to the shoulder, such as a fracture or dislocation. But sometimes the cause isn't well defined and instead the injury seems to emerge with the gradual wear and tear of age; like balding and gray hair, it can just happen.

Symptoms

If you injure your rotator cuff, you probably will have some of the following symptoms:

Rotator Cuff tear

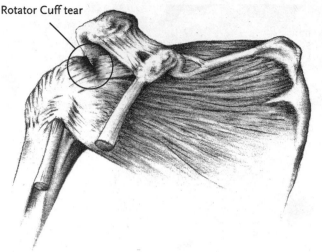

Typical anatomic findings associated with a rotator cuff tear.

Pain and tenderness in your shoulder, especially when reaching overhead. Pain is often localized to the deltoid muscle (which extends across the shoulder blade and helps raise the arm laterally) as well as the upper two-thirds of the arm. The pain can occasionally radiate down to the elbow. Numbness and tingling are usually not symptoms of rotator cuff problems, which include:

Difficulty sleeping on the affected side;

Shoulder weakness;

Shoulder stiffness;

Atrophy or thinning of the muscles around the shoulder;

Pain when you lower your arm from a fully raised position;

Crepitus (a crackling sensation) when you move your shoulder.

Diagnosis

Diagnosis of a rotator cuff tear will begin with a thorough examination. Your doctor will first check your shoulder for abnormalities. He or she should also palpate around your shoulder to see if there are any areas of tenderness, as well as measure the range of motion of your shoulder in several different directions and the strength of your arm. It is also important for your doctor to check for instability and problems with the acromioclavicular joint (the "knuckle" joint on the top of the shoulder)—and to examine your neck to make sure that your pain is not coming from a "pinched nerve" in your cervical spine or is a symptom of other conditions such as osteoarthritis or rheumatoid arthritis.

Imaging technologies are also used to diagnose rotator cuff injuries. But because X-rays of a shoulder with a rotator cuff tear are usually normal (or may show only a small spur), your doctor may find it useful to follow up with an MRI or even an ultrasound to better view this soft tissue area. In some circumstances an arthrogram—a radiographic study where a dye is injected into the joint before an X-ray is performed—may help your doctor evaluate your shoulder. Once a diagnosis of a rotator cuff tear has been made, your orthopedic surgeon will recommend one or more of a range of either nonsurgical or surgical treatments.

Nonsurgical Treatments
In most instances, nonsurgical methods can provide pain relief and can improve the function of your shoulder. These techniques may include:

RESTING THE SHOULDER. Stop doing what caused the pain and try to avoid painful movements. Limit heavy lifting or overhead activity until your shoulder feels better;

APPLYING ICE AND HEAT. Putting ice on your shoulder can help reduce inflammation and pain. Place a cold pack or a bag of frozen vegetables on the affected area for fifteen to twenty minutes every couple of hours during the first day or two. After about two or three days, when the pain and inflammation have subsided, applying hot packs or a heating pad may help relax your tight, sore muscles;

TAKING PAIN RELIEVERS. Over-the-counter acetaminophen (such as Tylenol) and nonsteroidal anti-inflammatory drugs (NSAIDs) such as aspirin, ibuprofen (such as Advil or Motrin) or naproxen (such as Aleve), may help reduce pain. Be sure first to discuss any medication treatment with your doctor, and stop taking the drugs when the pain improves;

KEEPING YOUR MUSCLES LIMBER. After one or two days, do some gentle exercises to keep your shoulder muscles flexible and loose;

RECEIVING STEROID INJECTIONS FROM YOUR PHYSICIAN. Doctors commonly inject steroids into the joint to relieve inflammation and pain. These have some side effects that include a low but serious risk of joint infection and, for diabetics, an elevation of blood sugar. (See Chapter 9 for detailed information about joint injections.)

Surgical Treatments

If there is no improvement after a sufficient period of time of conservative treatment (usually six to twelve weeks), your physician may consider surgery. (In some cases involving traumatic injury and significant impairment, surgical treatment may be warranted sooner.) In general, three approaches are available for surgical repair: arthroscopic repair, mini-open repair, and open surgical repair. During an arthroscopic repair, a fiber-optic scope and instruments are inserted through small puncture wounds instead of through an open incision. The scope is connected to a television monitor and the surgeon will perform the repair under video control. In a mini-open repair, surgeons perform a complete rotator cuff repair through an incision as small as two or three inches. And a traditional open surgical repair involves a larger incision but is often required if the tear itself is large or complicated.

In some severe cases, where arthritis has developed, shoulder replacement rather than repair is an option. Your surgeon will decide what approach is best for you based on your particular injury and circumstances.

General Tips for Prevention

Preventing rotator cuff tears involves following many of our same recommendations for avoiding other musculoskeletal injuries. In other words, you must practice common sense in your activities: always use good form; get into the habit of regularly exercising your rotator cuff; work on flexibility in your shoulder and throughout your body; and be careful not to stress your shoulder when you know that your overall conditioning is poor.

Exercises for Prevention and Healing

Most of the time, treatment after rotator cuff surgery involves exercise therapy, and, depending on the severity of your injury, this therapy may take from three weeks to several months to complete. Your surgeon will determine when you are ready to begin your therapy depending on the health of the surrounding muscles and tissues, the size of your tear, and the nature of the surgical repair. The following exercises may be among

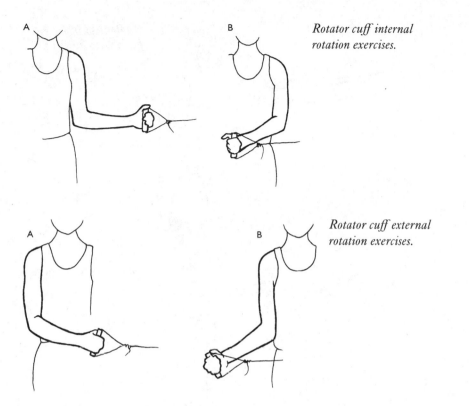

Rotator cuff internal rotation exercises.

Rotator cuff external rotation exercises.

those recommended by your surgeon. They use elastic tubing to increase strength and flexibility in the rotator cuff, and are designed to be done in two sets of ten movements each:

INTERNAL ROTATION. Grip some elastic tubing that is connected to a doorknob or other object at waist level. Keeping your elbow in at your side and your forearm parallel to the floor, rotate your arm inward across your body. Return your arm to the starting position and relax.

EXTERNAL ROTATION. Maintaining the same setup as for the internal rotation exercise, now face away from the door and, keeping your elbow in at your side, rotate your arm outward away from your body, making sure to keep your forearm parallel to the floor. Return your arm to the starting position and relax.

FLEXION. Face away from the door and, keeping your elbow straight, grasp the elastic tubing and pull your arm upward to

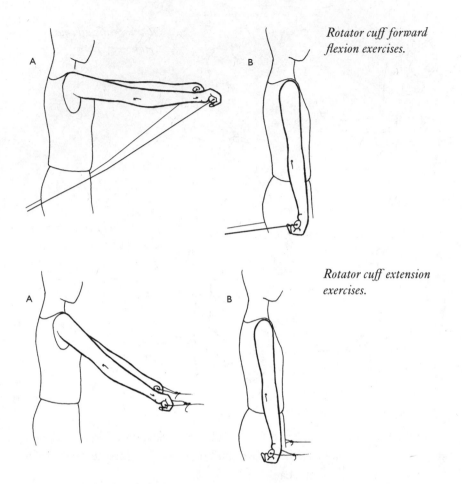

*Rotator cuff forward
flexion exercises.*

*Rotator cuff extension
exercises.*

shoulder height, or until you feel discomfort. Return your arm to
the starting position and relax.

EXTENSION. Face the door and, grasping the tubing, pull your arm
backward as high as you can comfortably reach. Be sure to keep
your elbow straight. Return your arm to the starting position and
relax.

LABRAL TEAR

The shoulder is made up of three bones: the scapula (shoulder blade), the
humerus (upper arm bone), and the clavicle (collarbone). A part of the scapula, called the glenoid, makes up the socket of the shoulder. The glenoid
is very shallow and flat, much like the tee in the golf ball analogy used
earlier in the chapter—so the shoulder joint would be relatively unstable

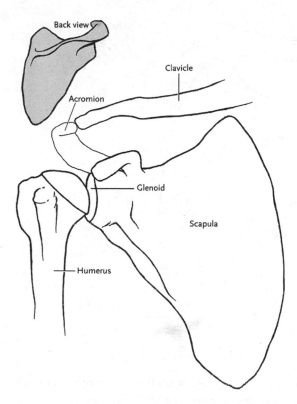

Back view

Clavicle

Acromion

Glenoid

Scapula

Humerus

The relationship between the clavicle, scapula, and humerus bones allows the shoulder to have the greatest range of motion of any joint in the body.

except for the labrum, a rim of soft tissue that makes the socket more like a cup.

The labrum adds stability and is exposed to a significant amount of stress. It is not surprising, then, that this rim often develops tears, particularly on the top part (or "superiorly")—hence the acronym SLAP ("superior labrum anterior posterior" tear). If the tear is extensive it may even cause a flap of tissue to move in and out of the joint, getting caught between the head of the humerus and the glenoid (in much the same way that a rug gets caught under a door). The flap can cause pain and a catching sensation when you move your shoulder. And because the biceps tendon (which originates in the big muscles on the front of your upper arm) and several ligaments attach to the labrum, when the labrum tears the shoulder often becomes less stable.

Causes

Sports can cause injuries to the labrum when the biceps tendon pulls sharply against the front of the labrum. Baseball pitchers are prone to

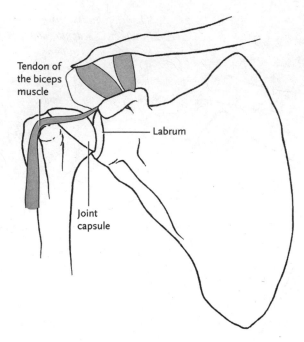

The relationship of the labrum to the biceps and humeral head.

Tendon of
the biceps
muscle

Labrum

Joint
capsule

labral tears because the action of throwing causes the biceps tendon to pull strongly against the top part of the labrum; weightlifters can have similar problems when pressing weights overhead. Golfers, too, may tear their labrum if their club strikes the ground during the golf swing, and volleyball players can injure their labrum when spiking a ball.

Other causes of labral tears include a fall on an outstretched hand that drives the humerus forcefully upward into the labrum, and a sudden and often unexpected load applied to the biceps, which adds undue stress on the labrum.

Symptoms

The main symptom of a labral tear is a sharp pop or catching sensation in the shoulder during certain shoulder movements. Although there may be a mild ache for several hours, the tear may not cause pain. In fact, any pain that you may feel is usually caused by inflammation of the capsule of the shoulder. Every time you move in a way that causes the labrum to flip back and forth, irritation and inflammation of the capsule occur. (For example, patients will often complain of pain when they try to reach into the back seat of a car while seated in the front.)

Diagnosis

Your doctor may suspect a labral tear based on how you injured your shoulder, so be ready to provide details about your most recent injury as well as information about any past damage to the area. In addition, he or she will conduct a physical examination and may challenge the shoulder with movements that can bring on the symptoms of a possible labral tear, perhaps raising the arm to see if you feel a catching sensation, or holding your arm briefly overhead to see if you experience pain when the shoulder is in that position.

Labral tears are difficult to see, even on an MRI, so doctors sometimes request an MRI arthrogram, in which dye is injected into the shoulder prior to performing the MRI in order to make the labrum more visible.

Treatments

Your doctor's first goal will be to control your pain and inflammation, so your initial treatment recommendation will likely be rest and anti-inflammatory medication such as acetaminophen or ibuprofen, as well as noninvasive techniques such as heat or ice. If anti-inflammatory medication doesn't control your pain, your doctor may suggest a cortisone injection (see Chapter 9 for details on these injections).

Rehabilitation will also be important, and your doctor will probably have a physical therapist direct your rehabilitation program. Hands-on manipulation of the muscles as well as various types of exercises will be employed to improve your range of motion in the shoulder and the nearby joints and muscles. Later in your recovery and treatment you will undertake strengthening exercises to improve the strength and control of the rotator cuff and shoulder blade muscles. Your therapist will assist you as you retrain these muscles to keep the ball of the humerus in the glenoid; doing so will improve the stability of your shoulder and help it move smoothly during all of your activities.

If you don't respond to conservative therapy, you may need surgery. Fortunately, the arthroscope can be used to treat many labral tears. If the tear is small and for the most part gets caught only as you move the shoulder, simply removing the frayed edges and any loose parts of the labrum (a process known as debridement) may get rid of your symptoms.

If the tear is larger, the shoulder may also be unstable. In this case, the labral tear may need to be repaired rather than simply removed. Several new techniques allow surgeons to place small anchors into the socket to help tack the labrum back down arthroscopically.

FROZEN SHOULDER

Adhesive capsulitis, or "frozen shoulder," is a disorder characterized by pain and loss of motion or stiffness in the shoulder. It affects about 2 percent of the general population and occurs most frequently in women between the ages of forty and seventy.

Causes

The causes of frozen shoulder are not fully understood but are thought to involve thickening and contracture of the capsule surrounding the shoulder joint. Frozen shoulder occurs much more commonly in people with diabetes, affecting 10 to 15 percent of diabetics. Other medical problems associated with increased risk of frozen shoulder include hypothyroidism (insufficient thyroid hormone levels in the blood), hyperthyroidism (excessive thyroid hormone levels in the blood), hypercholesterolemia (excessive blood cholesterol levels), and surgery (the exact reason for this is unknown). Frozen shoulder can also develop after a shoulder is injured or immobilized for an extended period.

Symptoms

The hallmark of the disorder is restricted motion or stiffness in the shoulder. The affected individual cannot move the shoulder normally, and motion is also limited when someone else attempts to move the shoulder for the patient. Pain due to frozen shoulder is usually dull or aching and becomes worse with attempted motion (especially when trying to reach over your head or behind your back). The pain is usually located in the outer shoulder area and sometimes in the upper arm.

Some physicians have described the normal course of a frozen shoulder as involving three stages. During the first, "freezing" stage, which may last from six weeks to nine months, the patient experiences a slow onset of pain. As the pain worsens, the shoulder loses motion. In the second stage, also called the "frozen" stage, the pain gradually lessens, but the stiffness remains. This stage generally lasts from four to nine months. During the third and final "thawing" stage, which generally lasts between five and twelve months, shoulder motion slowly returns to normal.

Diagnosis

As with many other joint disorders, diagnosis of a frozen shoulder is made by a physician after he or she inquires about symptoms and does a thorough medical exam. Imaging tests, such as X-rays or MRI, may be performed to rule out other possible causes for the loss of motion.

Treatments

The treatment of frozen shoulder is aimed at controlling pain and restoring motion. Pain control is usually achieved with anti-inflammatory medications; these include orally ingested pills such as ibuprofen or naproxyn, as well as injections such as corticosteroids. Narcotics should be avoided if at all possible because of the risk of addiction.

To regain motion, gentle physical therapy is usually started under the supervision of a therapist, and may be supplemented by a home exercise program designed by your physician or therapist. Physical therapy for this injury generally includes stretching or range-of-motion exercises for the shoulder; heat is sometimes used to help decrease pain. Attempts to strengthen the shoulder are generally not a good idea because doing so can exacerbate symptoms.

More than 90 percent of patients improve with these relatively simple treatments. In some cases, however, motion does not return completely and a small amount of stiffness remains even after several years. A good rule of thumb is that you can expect to regain 85 percent of your previous range of shoulder motion over time.

Surgery is considered when there is no improvement in pain or shoulder motion after six months of treatment involving physical therapy and anti-inflammatory medications. The most common surgeries for frozen shoulder include manipulation under anesthesia and shoulder arthroscopy with capsular release (which involves cutting the capsular tissue around the shoulder).

General Tips for Prevention

It is difficult to prevent frozen shoulder because it often accompanies systemic diseases like diabetes and thyroid disease—which are challenging to control. But you can help yourself achieve a complete recovery by beginning your prescribed range-of-motion exercises as soon after your shoulder injury as your physician will allow.

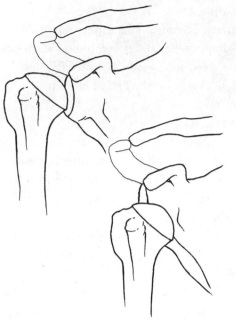

When a shoulder dislocates, it usually, but not always, comes out of the socket on the anterior side.

DISLOCATED SHOULDER

The shoulder joint is your body's most mobile major joint, allowing you to move your arm in many different directions. With such a range of motion comes an inherent instability of the joint, however, which can make it prone to dislocation—that is, a misplacement of adjacent bones.

Causes

Shoulder dislocations generally happen when a great deal of force is applied to the shoulder (usually suddenly). A dislocated shoulder may be caused by an impact during contact sports such as football and hockey or by a hard blow to your shoulder during a motor vehicle accident or a fall (perhaps while participating in a sport that involves frequent falls, such as downhill skiing, gymnastics, or volleyball). Dislocated shoulders are most common in people between the ages of fifteen and twenty-five because people in this age group tend to engage in a high level of physical activity.

While most shoulder dislocations occur in active individuals or are due to trauma, individuals whom we call loose jointed or double jointed are much more susceptible than others to shoulder dislocations. These patients have extreme flexibility and are naturally prone to dislocate; the amount of force needed to cause the shoulder to dislocate or slip out of the socket is less than that for most people. A trip to the emergency room is not usually required to reduce shoulder dislocations in these patients; instead they are diagnosed with "multidirectional instability" and are often best treated with shoulder strengthening exercises (not surgery).

Symptoms

Individuals who suspect a dislocated shoulder should seek prompt medical attention. When treated properly, most dislocated shoulders will return to near normal function after several weeks of rest and rehabilitation. Once you have experienced a dislocated shoulder, however, your joint may become prone to recurrent dislocations in the future. This is especially true if the first occurrence occurred between the ages of ten and thirty.

A dislocated shoulder joint is usually visibly deformed or out of place, swollen or discolored (bruised), intensely painful, and immovable. Shoulder dislocation may also cause numbness, weakness, or tingling near the injury, such as in your neck or down your arm. Additionally, the muscles in your shoulder may spasm from the disruption, which often increases the intensity of your pain.

Diagnosis

A physician should easily be able to diagnose a shoulder dislocation based on a detailed health and injury history as well as on a thorough physical examination of the shoulder. But a dislocated shoulder can sometimes cause muscles, ligaments, or tendons that reinforce your shoulder joint to tear; it can also cause bones (either the humerus or glenoid) to break. A dislocation can also occasionally lead to nerve or blood vessel damage around your shoulder joint, which can be a catastrophic injury. For this reason, further tests are usually ordered to rule out these serious complications. A diagnostic X-ray will be needed to assess the direction of the dislocation and evaluate whether an associated fracture of the shoulder is also present. In addition, an MRI may be done to help your doctor assess damage to the soft tissue structures around your shoulder joint after the shoulder is relocated. For example, with older patients the rotator cuff can often be torn due to a shoulder dislocation. Younger patients are more likely to tear the cartilage ring around the shoulder (labrum). As part of the X-ray or MRI process, an arthrogram may be performed, which involves injecting a fluid into your shoulder to highlight certain structures of your shoulder joint. If your shoulder has been dislocated, the fluid may leak into an area of your shoulder joint where it normally would not be found, indicating a tear or abnormal opening such as those caused by ligament damage.

Any nerve damage would be discovered through the use of electromyography (EMG), which is a test (not a very fun one because it involves a number of needles) that measures the electrical discharges produced in your muscles.

If bones, ligaments, or tendons in your shoulder have been damaged, or if nerves or blood vessels surrounding your shoulder joint have been injured, you may need surgery.

Nonsurgical Treatments

In general, traumatic dislocations require a trip to the emergency room, where a physician will administer pain medication and realign the joint into its proper position. This realignment should be performed by a physician only, and he or she will try various maneuvers to help your shoulder bones get back where they belong. Depending on the amount of pain and swelling, you may need a muscle relaxant or sedative or, rarely, a general anesthetic before your shoulder bones can be manipulated in this way.

After your shoulder is put back into its proper position, your pain should ease immediately. Complete pain relief, however, will not occur until the joint swelling resolves (usually after a few days). Your doctor may put your shoulder in a special splint or sling for several weeks; how long you wear it will depend on the nature of your shoulder dislocation. Your doctor may also prescribe a pain reliever to keep you comfortable during the first few days of healing.

Recent studies by Dr. Eiji Itoi in Japan have shown that putting the shoulder in the external rotation position (with the elbow at the side and the forearm extending outward from the body, with thumb up) may help reduce recurrence after a dislocation. But it has been difficult to persuade patients to fix their arms in such an awkward position, and so far the technique has not caught on in the United States.

If you've experienced a fairly simple shoulder dislocation without major nerve or tissue damage, your shoulder joint will likely return to normal (although recurrent dislocations are possible). Problems arise if your shoulder keeps dislocating, because each time your shoulder dislocates there is more damage to your soft tissue, cartilage, and bone. Depending on the extent of this damage, a relatively simple surgical procedure can be turned into a complex surgical reconstruction that can result in premature arthritis.

Surgical Treatments

If your doctor cannot move your dislocated shoulder bones back into position by manipulating them from outside of your body, he will need to use open methods (surgery) to do so. In addition, even if your shoulder is easily put back into place, you may need to have surgery to correct any serious damage to the shoulder joint or to ligaments—damage that would likely lead to recurring shoulder dislocations (shoulder instability).

Surgery may be arthroscopic (camera-guided) or open. The surgical method used depends on the extent of the injury, the demands placed on the shoulder by the patient, and the surgeon's skill and preference. Each technique has pros and cons that your surgeon should discuss with you; the techniques differ in terms of pain during recovery, length of recovery, and likelihood of success. In general, whereas arthroscopic surgery can generally be done on an outpatient basis, you will have to wait a bit longer to return to your normal activities because the repair is not as robust as when you have open surgery. But open surgery can have its own drawbacks. Surprisingly, one of the risks of surgery—especially open surgery—is overtightening of the shoulder joint, which results in excessive stiffness in the shoulder that can eventually lead to arthritis. Although some stiffness in the shoulder is to be expected, too much can be problematic and may even require a repeat surgery.

SHOULDER ARTHRITIS

Arthritis of the shoulder is a painful condition that affects one or both of the two joints that make up the shoulder. Shoulder arthritis typically affects patients over fifty years old and is most common in patients with prior shoulder injuries.

Causes

Shoulder arthritis is often caused by wear and tear associated with age (that is, osteoarthritis), but it can also accompany rheumatoid arthritis or arthritis that occurs after a fracture, dislocation, or other trauma.

Symptoms

Several symptoms characterize shoulder arthritis:

- Pain in the shoulder that increases during activity and becomes progressively worse over time
- Pain that increases with changes in the weather

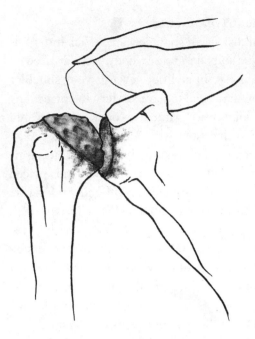

An osteoarthritic shoulder, showing typical loss of cartilage, bone spur formation, and joint space narrowing.

- Limited shoulder motion

- A clicking or snapping sound as the shoulder is moved

Diagnosis

To diagnose arthritis of the shoulder, your doctor will usually rely on a detailed history of the injury and of the trouble you are currently experiencing, as well as a careful physical exam of the shoulder. In addition, he or she will probably order an X-ray or MRI to help rule out other possible sources of the problem.

Nonsurgical Treatments

There are several nonsurgical treatments that a physician may prescribe depending on the seriousness of the arthritis and the amount of pain:

- Activity modification

- Anti-inflammatory medication

- Corticosteroid injections (see Chapter 9 for details)

- Physical therapy (although because traditional physical therapy can occasionally aggravate the symptoms, aquatic therapy may be preferred)

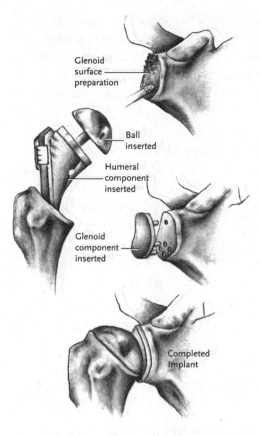

Glenoid
surface
preparation

Ball
inserted

Humeral
component
inserted

Glenoid
component
inserted

Completed
Implant

Shoulder replacement involves resurfacing the socket with a plastic liner and replacing the humeral head with a metal sphere.

Surgical Treatment Options

If the nonsurgical options do not work, or if the problem is serious, surgery may be recommended. Shoulder replacement is generally the gold standard treatment for shoulder arthritis, because arthroscopy of the shoulder for this problem tends to be of limited benefit. Total shoulder replacement is believed to provide the most predictable postoperative pain relief for patients with osteoarthritis of the shoulder. In shoulder replacement, a surgeon replaces or resurfaces the shoulder joint using metal and plastic components. The humeral component is made of metal, usually a combination of a chrome-cobalt head with a titanium stem; the glenoid component is most commonly made of ultra-high-molecular-weight polyethylene. Shoulder replacement surgery, much like hip and knee replacement, is generally very successful.

General Tips for Prevention

Arthritis of the shoulder is very difficult to avoid because it usually develops in concert with other conditions that are hard to overcome. But it can be helpful to learn which activities may strain the shoulder (and to avoid them), as well as to do some flexibility exercises at home if your doctor approves.

Exercises for Prevention and Healing

Gentle physical therapy is usually started under the supervision of a therapist and may be supplemented by a home exercise program designed by your physician or therapist. Physical therapy can generally include stretching or range-of-motion exercises for the shoulder as well as mild strengthening; heat is sometimes used to help decrease pain. Aggressive strengthening exercises are generally not a good idea because doing so can exacerbate symptoms. Much like when you have a pebble in your shoe, arthritis can be made more painful with excessive activity.

MAIN POINTS TO REMEMBER

- The shoulder is a versatile but delicate joint—be careful not to misuse it

- Unlike treatment options for many joint injuries, those for frozen shoulder do not include strengthening exercises

- Dislocations of the shoulder frequently involve additional injuries to the surrounding muscles, ligaments, bones, and tendons

- Shoulder arthritis, while not as common as hip and knee arthritis, has similar treatment options: activity modification, anti-inflammatory medication, periodic cortisone injections, and, when all else fails, joint replacement.

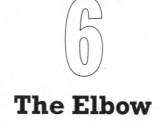

The Elbow

IT'S HARD TO IMAGINE LIFE without the use of the elbow, the joint where three long bones meet in the middle of your arm and allow you to do essential, enjoyable tasks like hugging a friend, feeding yourself, and swinging a baseball bat. There the bone of the upper arm (humerus) connects to both the inner bone of the forearm (ulna) and the outer bone of the forearm (radius) to form a hinge joint. The inner and outer forearm bones also themselves connect in the elbow, allowing the forearm to rotate.

Muscles are a vital component of the elbow joint. The biceps and brachialis muscles are the main elbow flexors, while the triceps extends the elbow. Some tendons of the elbow attach to the bony bump along the outer elbow, called the lateral epicondyle, which is part of the humerus bone. These tendons can be injured, causing inflammation or tendonitis (lateral epicondylitis, or "tennis elbow"). Other tendons attach to the bony bump along the inside of the elbow, called the medial epicondyle; tendons that attach here also can become inflamed and injured, causing medial epicondylitis, or "golfer's elbow." A fluid-filled sac (bursa), which helps reduce friction, overlies the tip of the elbow and also can become inflamed in a condition known as olecranon bursitis.

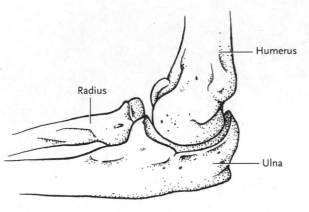

The elbow involves intricate relationships among the humerus, radius, and ulna.

Radius

Humerus

Ulna

TENNIS ELBOW

Tennis elbow, or lateral epicondylitis, is a degenerative condition of the tendon fibers that attach to the bony prominence on the outside of the elbow. The tendons involved are responsible for anchoring the muscles that extend or lift the wrist and hand as well as supinate the hand (turn the palm upward).

Causes

Tennis elbow is brought on by:

- Tight or weak forearm muscles

- The use of faulty arm motions in racquet sports and weightlifting

- Overuse of the elbow in sports such as tennis, racquetball, squash, or fencing

- Overuse of the elbow in activities such as meat cutting, painting, raking, or weaving

- A sudden increase in the intensity of a workout or sports activity

- Overuse of the elbow in certain professions such as plumbing, car repair, and carpentry

Tennis elbow happens mostly in patients between the ages of thirty and fifty, although it can occur at any age. The syndrome can affect as many as half the number of athletes who participate in racquet sports, but interestingly most patients with tennis elbow are not active in these sports. While most of the time no specific traumatic injury occurs before the symptoms

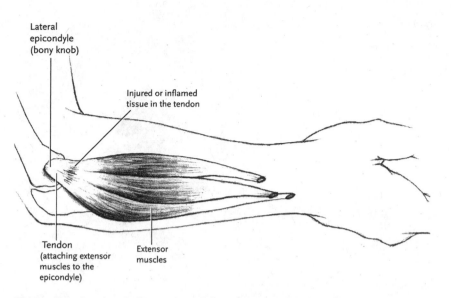

Lateral
epicondyle
(bony knob)

Injured or inflamed
tissue in the tendon

Tendon
(attaching extensor
muscles to the
epicondyle)

Extensor
muscles

Tennis elbow involves inflammation of the extensor tendons located on the outer aspect of the elbow.

arise, many individuals with tennis elbow are involved in work or recreational activities that require repetitive and vigorous use of the forearm muscles.

Symptoms

Patients often complain of severe, burning pain on the outer part of the elbow. In most cases, the pain is rather mild at first but gradually increases over weeks to months. The pain can be made worse by performing a back-hand stroke in racquet sports, golfing, turning a doorknob, weightlifting, pressing on the outer part of the elbow, or gripping or lifting objects, especially with the palm facing down. Even lifting light objects such as a book or a cup of coffee can cause significant discomfort. In more severe cases, pain can occur with simple movement of the elbow and radiate to the forearm.

Diagnosis

Your doctor may press on various parts of your elbow and ask you to lift your wrist or fingers against resistance to see whether your lateral epicondyle is injured. X-rays are usually not necessary to diagnose tennis elbow. Rarely MRI scans may be used to show changes in the tendon where it attaches to bone.

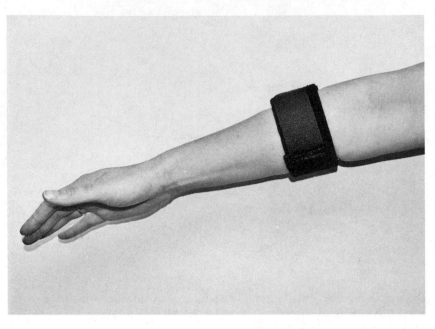

A counterforce strap or clasp is often used to decrease the inflammation associated with tennis elbow.

Nonsurgical Treatments

Treatment of tennis elbow involves rest and avoiding those activities that worsen your pain. The use of counterforce straps can help with symptoms; these rest the muscles and tendons of your elbow and should provide significant pain relief within four to six weeks.

In mild cases of tennis elbow, nonsteroidal anti-inflammatory agents may be helpful. Injection of corticosteroids and a local anesthetic into the painful area may also be of assistance in cases that don't respond to conservative therapy, although an excessive number of injections should be avoided due to possible local and systemic side effects of steroids. Your physician may recommend physical therapy, which would probably involve stretching and range-of-motion exercises, as well as gradual strengthening of the affected muscles and tendons. Thankfully, nonoperative treatment is successful in as many as 90 percent of tennis elbow cases.

After the pain has resolved, a daily physical therapy program involving stretching of the tendons may be helpful. Consulting a professional about your playing technique and the grip size on your racket may also prevent recurrence.

A new treatment called extracorporeal shock wave therapy (ESWT) is also being applied to tennis elbow in some clinics, although its use is somewhat controversial. The treatment uses sound waves to cause tissues to experience microtrauma, which is thought to initiate a healing response and help decrease the inflammation that characterizes tennis elbow. Shock waves are also used in the treatment of heel spurs and kneecap tendonitis. If you are diagnosed with tennis elbow, you may want to ask your doctor whether this new therapy might provide some relief.

Surgical Treatments

Surgery is considered only for those patients who have incapacitating pain that does not respond to nonoperative therapy. Surgery for tennis elbow involves removing diseased tendon tissue and reattaching normal tendon tissue to bone. The surgery is usually performed through a small incision over the bony prominence of the outer elbow, although some centers are now performing this outpatient procedure through an arthroscope. A splint is placed on the elbow for a week, after which exercises to stretch the elbow and restore range of motion are started. Strengthening exercises are begun gradually two months after surgery, and most people can resume their athletic activity within four to six months. Tennis elbow surgery is successful for approximately 90 percent of patients.

Exercises for Prevention and Healing

Many of the muscles and tendons that become overused and cause tennis elbow can be trained to be more flexible and thus resistant to trauma. The following exercises are designed to give you ways to stretch, warm up, and strengthen these parts of the elbow:

> BACKHAND STRETCH. Hold your arm out in front of you, keeping your elbow straight and the palm of your palm face down. Reach with your other hand and press the back of your extended hand gently downward until you feel a stretch on the back of your forearm. Hold for ten seconds and release.

> FOREHAND STRETCH. Hold your arm out in front of you, keeping your elbow straight and the palm of your hand face down. With your other hand lift the fingertips of your extended hand slowly up and back until you feel a gentle stretch along the palm side of your wrist and forearm. Hold for ten seconds and release.

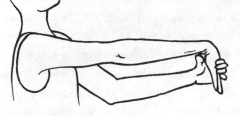

Backhand stretch.

BACKHAND LIFT. Sit with your injured elbow relaxed and bent at 90 degrees with the palm down on your thigh. Slowly bend your wrist upward as far as you can without causing pain. Hold for two counts, then slowly lower back to the original position. Add a maximum of one pound of weight (held in the palm of your hand) if you can do this exercise completely without pain.

WRIST ROTATION. Sit with your injured elbow bent at 90 degrees and your hand resting palm up on your knee. Hold a one to two pound weight in your hand. Slowly rotate your palm down, and then up, lifting the weight slightly above your knee.

"THUMB'S UP." Sit with your injured elbow straight, hand resting on your knee and your thumb pointing up. Slowly bend your wrist up as far as possible without lifting it. Hold for two counts, then slowly lower your wrist and relax. You can try adding up to one pound of weight, as long as you do not experience any pain.

GOLFER'S ELBOW

Golfer's elbow (medial epicondylitis), like tennis elbow, is caused by overuse of the muscles and tendons of the forearm. But whereas tennis elbow primarily affects the extensors of the wrist and hand (the muscles and tendons that extend the wrist and hand to its straightened position), golfer's elbow afflicts the flexor pronator muscles of the inner elbow—that is, those muscles and tendons that allow the wrist and forearm to flex and rotate.

Causes

Golfer's elbow may be caused by a single violent action; more commonly, however, it develops over time as a muscle is overused in a narrowly repetitive way. Golfer's elbow occurs more commonly at the beginning of

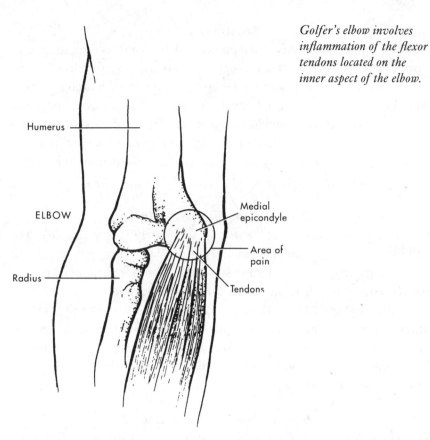

Golfer's elbow involves inflammation of the flexor tendons located on the inner aspect of the elbow.

Humerus

ELBOW

Radius

Medial epicondyle

Area of pain

Tendons

the golf season, when the muscles and tendons are suddenly used in a more intense and/or constant way. Similarly, when other activities that can cause golfer's elbow (such as woodworking or sports other than golf) are suddenly done more intensively or frequently, medial epicondylitis can result.

Symptoms

The pain of golfer's elbow is usually limited to the elbow area; some patients, however, also experience a shooting sensation down the forearm when they grip objects.

Diagnosis

A physician will examine your elbow closely and ask questions about your activities and any injuries. Rarely, imaging technologies such as X-rays or MRI scans will be needed to confirm the initial diagnosis.

Treatments

Medial epicondylitis is usually a limited problem that does not cause long-term disability. A little rest and proper rehabilitation are usually effective treatments, and surgery is rarely necessary. Patients with golfer's elbow should avoid the offending activity until the pain has subsided; once the pain is gone, the activity should be reinstated only gradually. RICE therapy (rest, ice, compression, and elevation) can decrease inflammation following the activity, as can taking a nonsteroidal anti-inflammatory medication such as ibuprofen.

General Tips for Prevention

It is important to stretch and warm up adequately before and after the activity that caused your elbow injury. On the days when you are resting from that activity, you may want to strengthen your forearm muscles with exercises like those listed here. (Most fitness stores sell resistance elastic bands that can be used to work the muscles of the forearm as well.) If these simple measures do not help, your physician may recommend a series of cortisone injections into the area. Surgery, if needed, would be aimed at decreasing the tension on the tendons that are inflamed and can be done on an outpatient basis.

Exercises for Prevention and Healing

To avoid golfer's elbow, the American Academy of Orthopaedic Surgeons suggests these simple exercises to help build up your forearm muscles:

SQUEEZING A TENNIS BALL. Squeezing a tennis ball in your hand for five minutes at a time is a simple, effective exercise to strengthen your forearm muscles.

WRIST CURLS WITH A LIGHTWEIGHT DUMBBELL. Hold one arm out in front of you, bent at 90 degrees. With your palm up, lower the weight to the end of your fingers, then curl the weight back into your palm; curl up your wrist only to lift the weight an inch or two higher. Do ten repetitions with one arm before repeating with the other arm.

REVERSE WRIST CURLS. With your hand in front of you, palm down, lift a lightweight dumbbell up and down with your wrist. With the nonexercising hand, hold the upper arm of your exercising arm in order to limit motion in the exercising forearm. Do ten repetitions with one arm before switching to and repeating with the other arm.

ARTHRITIS OF THE ELBOW

An often very painful condition, arthritis of the elbow occurs when the cartilage surface of the elbow is damaged or becomes worn.

Causes

Sometimes the wear or damage that causes arthritis of the elbow can be traced to a previous injury (for example, a dislocation of the elbow or a fracture linked to age-related degeneration of the joint cartilage). Although osteoarthritis commonly affects weight-bearing joints like the hip and knee, the elbow can also be afflicted.

Most patients with elbow osteoarthritis have a history of injury to the elbow (such as a fracture or dislocation). The risk for elbow arthritis increases if surgery was required to repair the injury or reconstruct the joint; if joint cartilage has been lost; or if the joint surface was unable to be repaired or reconstructed to its preinjury level. Significantly, an injury to the ligaments that results in an unstable elbow can also lead to arthritis because any imbalance or change in how the elbow moves and absorbs shock will often cause the joint to wear out more rapidly.

Elbow arthritis does not have to be caused by an isolated traumatic injury; work or recreational activities may also lead to elbow arthritis if the patient places more demands on the joint than it can bear. Baseball pitchers, for example, place unusually high demands on their throwing elbows that can lead to failure of the stabilizing ligaments. The high shear forces placed across the joint during activities like throwing or playing a racquet sport can lead to cartilage breakdown over a period of years.

Symptoms

The most common symptoms of elbow arthritis are pain and/or loss of range of motion; in addition, patients usually complain of a "grating" or "locking" sensation in the elbow. The "grating," or rough rubbing sensation, is due to loss of the normal smooth joint surface and is caused by cartilage damage or wear; the "locking" is caused by loose pieces of cartilage or bone that can dislodge from the joint and become trapped between the moving joint surfaces, blocking motion.

In later stages, patients might also notice numbness in their ring and small fingers caused by elbow swelling or limited range of motion. The tingling occurs because the "funny bone" (ulnar nerve) is located in a tight tunnel behind the inner (medial) side of the elbow, and swelling in the elbow joint can put increased pressure on the nerve.

Diagnosis

A doctor can usually diagnose elbow arthritis based on a patient's symptoms and on standard X-rays. Most of the time, advanced imaging studies such as CT or MRI scans are not needed. Elbow osteoarthritis that occurs without previous injury is more common in men than in women, and usually begins after age fifty.

Nonsurgical Treatments

Treatment will depend on the stage of the arthritis, prior history of injury, the patient's wishes, the patient's medical condition, and X-ray findings. Early stages of elbow arthritis are treated medically with oral medications such as acetaminophen or ibuprofen, physical therapy, activity modification, and joint injections. In particular, steroid injections can provide significant relief, and injection of hyaluronic acid, a process called viscosupplementation, can also be attempted to increase the fluid in the joint and to "cushion" the diseased cartilage (see Chapter 9 for details).

Surgical Treatments

By the time arthritis can be seen on X-rays, the joint surfaces have already become significantly worn. If the damage is limited, arthroscopy (camera-guided surgery) can offer a minimally invasive surgical treatment. Arthroscopy involves removing free-floating debris or damaged tissues in the joint while smoothing out irregular surfaces. Multiple small incisions are used. By contrast, if the joint surface of the elbow has worn away completely, joint replacement may be required. For those patients who need this invasive surgery, dramatic pain relief and improvement in function can occur. But this alternative is generally offered only to elderly patients who place low demands on their elbows because the replacement options for the elbow are still not as durable as those for the hip, knee, and shoulder.

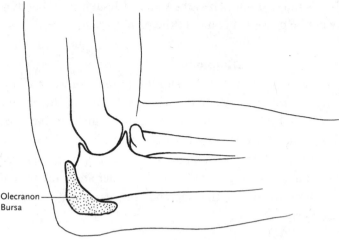

In olecranon bursitis, the bursa on the back of the elbow becomes inflamed and fluid-filled.

Olecranon Bursa

OLECRANON BURSITIS

The olecranon bursa is a sac of fluid that lies on the back of the elbow to allow for smooth movement of the joint. Olecranon bursitis, a common cause of swelling and pain around the elbow, occurs when the olecranon bursa becomes inflamed and the sac fills with additional fluid.

Causes

Olecranon bursitis may follow a traumatic accident such as landing on the elbow during a fall onto a hard floor or artificial turf. People who rest their elbows on hard surfaces—for example on a desktop while writing—may also cause or aggravate the condition and make the swelling more prominent. A systemic inflammatory process (such as rheumatoid arthritis), or a disease that involves the depositing of crystals within the body (for example, gout or pseudogout) can also trigger olecranon bursitis—and may be suspected if inflammation is present at other sites in the body. The swelling and inflammation can occasionally be the result of an infection within the bursa.

Symptoms

The hallmarks of olecranon bursitis are pain and a noticeable swelling at the bony part of the elbow. The pain usually worsens with pressure, such as when you lean on your elbow, and you may find that you bump the swollen elbow frequently because it protrudes farther than normal.

Usually the elbow's range of motion is the same, although fully bending your elbow may not be possible because of the pain.

Diagnosis

Your doctor can diagnose olecranon bursitis by examining your elbow and by what he learns from having you describe the history of the trouble with your elbow (as well as whether you participate in any activities that may have caused or worsened your symptoms). If you have a lot of pain while performing range-of-motion tests, or if your symptoms occurred after a traumatic injury, your doctor will probably order an X-ray to find out whether you have a fracture of the olecranon process (the protruding, bony part of the elbow).

Treatments

Treatment for routine olecranon bursitis typically involves changing the way you use your elbow and taking over-the-counter nonsteroidal anti-inflammatory medicine. Sometimes drainage of the fluid from the olecranon bursa is required, a procedure that may be followed by an injection of cortisone into the inflamed sac in order to suppress the inflammatory response for a longer period. Analysis of the drained fluid can determine whether an active infection is present (if an infection is detected, antibiotic therapy will be prescribed). In the absence of infection, most patients respond very well to conservative treatment and perhaps an additional one or two sessions of draining the fluid, with or without an accompanying corticosteroid injection. Although the inflammation typically subsides after resting the elbow and draining the fluid as needed, patients will often feel a pebblelike bump of thickened bursa many months after suffering from an episode of olecranon bursitis. Rarely, if the bursitis returns persistently, the bursa will need to be surgically removed.

You can help your olecranon bursa heal more quickly by taking some simple measures at home.

During the first two to five days after the injury, ice the posterior elbow for fifteen to twenty minutes several times a day;

Compress the elbow using an elastic wrap or sleeve;

Avoid excessive pressure on or around the elbow;

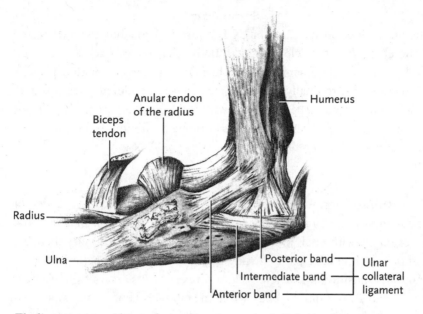

Anular tendon
of the radius

Biceps
tendon

Humerus

Radius

Ulna

Posterior band
Intermediate band — Ulnar
collateral
Anterior band — ligament

The ligamentous and bony relationships seen on the medial side of a normal elbow.

Avoid situations that may lead to further trauma of the area;

Consider using elbow pads to cushion the region.

If you have a problem with recurrent buildup of fluid in the bursa, ask your doctor whether you should use a posterior plaster splint to limit elbow motion for one to two weeks after the fluid is drained.

ULNAR COLLATERAL LIGAMENT INJURY

The ulnar collateral ligament (UCL) is essential for stabilizing the elbow and for this reason plays an important role in most throwing sports such as baseball and javelin, as well as in racquet sports and ice hockey.

Causes

Repetitive throwing motions in athletes are the most common cause of UCL injury, although traumatic valgus stress to the elbow during a fall or with the arm outstretched can also lead to UCL rupture (often with an accompanying elbow dislocation).

Symptoms

The most common symptom of UCL injury is pain along the medial side of the elbow (the side closest to the body) that is most acute during an overhead throw. The pain is often chronic or recurrent, with a player's throwing ability gradually affected; or it can occur suddenly, perhaps during a single throw, and be associated with a popping sensation. Swelling or bruising can be a problem, and a loss of range of motion in the elbow also can occur occasionally.

Diagnosis

Along with asking you about the pain and any traumatic injury, your doctor may request that you try particular movements with your arm and elbow. For example, with UCL injuries, pain may be elicited with a clenched fist. And pain and possible joint opening can occur when the doctor puts your elbow in a position that elicits valgus stress (valgus refers to movement of the hand away from the body while the elbow is kept in the same position) or with the elbow in 25 degrees of flexion (elbow abduction stress test). The affected side can be compared with the outer part of the same elbow to determine if there are significant differences in how loose the joint appears. (Documenting baseline elbow laxity in elite athletes, especially pitchers, before the season begins may be helpful for comparison if an injury occurs during the season, because some throwing athletes are asymmetrical from the start.)

Although ordinary X-rays can, in some cases, reveal ligament ossification and other symptoms suggestive of UCL injuries, as well as rule out other causes of elbow pain, MRI with its sharp contrast is rapidly becoming the imaging technique of choice for documenting ligament rupture (much as it is for all soft tissue injuries).

Nonsurgical Treatments

If you are diagnosed with damage to the UCL, your doctor will most likely recommend three to six months of conservative physical therapy, along with rest, nonsteroidal anti-inflammatory drugs (NSAIDs), and exercises to improve the elbow's range of motion. Only after the range of motion is restored and the pain and swelling are gone will you be able to return to your throwing activity, as long as you increase only gradually the velocity of your throwing and the duration of your training sessions.

Surgical Treatments

Surgical repair is generally indicated for acute tears in competitive athletes when instability exists, or when the patient has recurring pain and looseness in the joint after two or more attempts at conservative therapy. Reconstruction of the UCL is usually performed using a graft from one's own tendons (the palmaris longus, which extends along the forearm, is often used) or from a donor tendon. Consultation with an orthopedic surgeon, preferably a sports or upper extremity specialist, is recommended when surgery is being considered. Note that steroid injection is generally not recommended for UCL injuries.

General Tips for Prevention

Flexibility and strength training of the elbow can help prevent recurrent injury to the UCL. In addition, it is essential to evaluate your throwing technique with the goal of preventing reinjury during the healing phase as well as after normal training is resumed. You shouldn't participate in competitive sports involving throwing until you no longer experience pain while throwing; your elbow and shoulder range of motion return to near normal; your forearm strength is restored; and you have established a good throwing technique that will not cause further injury.

Exercises for Prevention and Healing

If you are a throwing athlete, your throwing activities will usually be limited for approximately six to eight weeks following the injury. The actual length of rest depends on the severity of the soreness. In approximately seven to ten days, you may begin a light stretching program under the direction of your doctor or physical therapist. The stretches should include the wrist flexors, wrist extensors, and elbow flexors. In addition, you will probably begin a light strengthening program. You should start with isometric strengthening and perform these exercises for one week. Then, at three weeks, if your doctor and physical therapist agree, you may begin the commonly prescribed Thrower's Ten exercise program (ask your doctor or therapist for details). Once you have full and pain-free range of motion, normal strength, and no tenderness over the injured area, you may begin an interval-throwing program again under the direction of a physician or physical therapist. If you are a throwing athlete, you should begin throwing from short distances and gradually increase the distance over several weeks.

MAIN POINTS TO REMEMBER

- Overuse of the elbow—during sports, work, or other activities—can lead to injury

- Although osteoarthritis commonly affects the weight-bearing joints, it can also afflict the elbow

- The replacement options for the elbow are not as advanced as they are for other joints such as the shoulder, hip, and knee

- Exercising your forearms to increase flexibility and strength in the muscles and ligaments supporting the elbow can help to prevent tennis elbow and golfer's elbow

7

The Hand and Wrist

THE HAND AND WRIST ARE among the most complex and important parts of the human body. We rely on our hands, with their nimble opposable thumbs—and our wrists, with their finely tuned tendons, ligaments, and bones—to help us work, care for others, lift and catch objects, drive, and complete the myriad other tasks of our day with precision and sensitivity. Because we are so dependent on our hands and wrists, injuries to these areas can have a tremendous influence on our quality of life. But caring for such intricate parts of the body is not easy. The hand and wrist are composed of no fewer than twenty-seven bones, including the eight carpal bones in the wrist, five metacarpal bones that form the palm of the hand, and fourteen phalanges—small bones that, when strung together, form the thumb and fingers.

WRIST SPRAIN
Wrist sprains are traumatic injuries to the ligaments and tendons support-ing the wrist joint.

Causes
Wrist sprains commonly occur when people instinctively put one or both hands out to try and break their falls, then land hard on their palms, jam-

ming or twisting their wrists. Wrist sprains are also common occurrences in sporting activities such as football, basketball, volleyball, skiing, and ice skating. Sprains of the wrist are graded according to the severity of the injury, with Grade 1 injuries being mild and Grade 3 severe.

Symptoms

The most characteristic symptoms of wrist sprains are swelling around the wrist joint, pain upon moving the wrist, and bruising or discoloration of the skin.

Diagnosis

Your physician will make a diagnosis after examining your wrist and questioning you about how the injury occurred. You will likely need to have your wrist X-rayed to definitively rule out a fracture within the many interconnected bones of the wrist; an MRI scan is rarely necessary but can sometimes be helpful if your diagnosis is unclear or if the symptoms do not improve.

Treatments

Treatment of a sprained wrist follows the RICE method—rest, ice, compression, and elevation—tailored for injuries in this area:

> REST. Use your wrist sparingly for the first day or two after your injury; avoid any activities that cause pain. You may want to purchase an over-the-counter wrist splint to protect your wrist.

> ICE. Ice the sprained wrist for twenty minutes every three to four hours for the first two days after your injury.

> COMPRESSION. Using an Ace bandage, wrap the wrist from the base of the fingers all the way to the top of the forearm, making sure it is not wrapped so tightly as to cut off your circulation.

> ELEVATION. Keep your sprained wrist elevated.

General Tips for Prevention

Protective gear for certain sports can reduce the risk of sustaining a wrist sprain.

Wrist Symptoms That Require Medical Attention

• Deformity of the wrist after injury

• Signs of a wrist infection, including fever, pain, swelling, redness, or warmth

• Wrist pain at night or while at rest

• Swelling and bruising around the wrist or forearm

• Inability to carry objects or use the wrist

• Wrist pain for more than three to five days

• Inability to bend and straighten the wrist

TENDONITIS OF THE HAND OR WRIST

Tendonitis is an inflammation of a tendon. In the wrist, the flexor tendons are on the palm side of the wrist and hand, whereas the extensor tendons occupy the back of the wrist and hand. These hand and wrist tendons pass through distinct compartments either individually or in groups; when the tendons become irritated, their ability to glide within these compartments can become limited. This impairment can then lead to hand and wrist pain during movement or when pressure is applied.

Causes

The hand and wrist tendons can become injured from excessive or unconditioned use or from direct trauma; when this occurs, the sheath lining them becomes inflamed and movements become painful as the tendons fail to glide easily through the sheath.

One example of an unconditioned use is when a person engages in a strenuous activity only occasionally: for example, someone who skis only infrequently can easily develop tendonitis in the extensor tendons in the wrist from gripping the ski pole during a several-day ski trip.

Symptoms

If you have wrist tendonitis, your wrist will hurt when you repeat the motion that caused the injury, and your wrist area will be tender to the

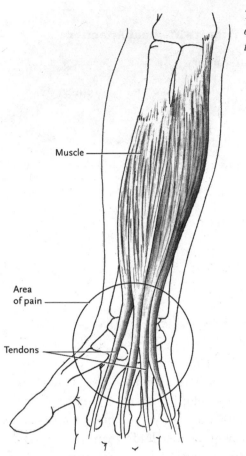

Tendonitis of the wrist can involve one of many tendons that cross over the wrist joint.

Muscle

Area
of pain

Tendons

touch. In more severe cases, the tendon will become so inflamed that it will produce a crackling noise as it moves within the sheath; there may also be redness and swelling.

Diagnosis

Your doctor can usually make a diagnosis of wrist tendonitis based on the history you provide and on a simple examination. Unless the physician is worried about associated injuries, no other studies (such as ultrasound, X-rays, or MRIs) will likely be needed.

Nonsurgical Treatments

Treatment of wrist tendonitis typically involves rest, immobilization, and anti-inflammatory medication. For most patients, this therapy will eliminate their symptoms in two to three weeks, but some will be unable to modify their activities due to work or family responsibilities, such as having a young child they need to carry. For example, new mothers who develop DeQuervain's tenosynovitis—a tendonitis of the extensor tendons caused by suddenly having to hold a child all the time—may take much longer to heal because it is nearly impossible for them to avoid lifting and carrying a baby under their care.

Surgical Treatments

Surgery is performed only when all other treatments have failed to alleviate the symptoms. Surgery for wrist tendonitis involves cutting open the tight tendon sheath that causes the painful and difficult tendon movements.

CARPAL TUNNEL SYNDROME

The median nerve travels from the forearm into the hand through a somewhat narrow passageway in your wrist called the carpal tunnel. The bottom and sides of this tunnel are formed by wrist bones, and the top is covered by a thick band of connective tissue. In addition to the median nerve, this tunnel also contains nine tendons. Carpal tunnel syndrome (CTS) is the condition that results from compression of the median nerve as it passes through the wrist.

Causes

Because so many tendons share this tight space with the median nerve, a variety of conditions and physical activities can cause compression of the nerve and result in symptoms such as numbness, tingling in the hand, clumsiness, or pain. These include: systemic problems such as diabetes, alcohol abuse, thyroid disease, pregnancy, and arthritis (particularly rheumatoid arthritis); repetitive overuse of the hand and wrist (perhaps at the computer keyboard); increased intensity and duration of wrist-dependent exercise such as racket sports; improper or ill-fitting sports equipment; broken or dislocated bones in the wrist that produce swelling; or being over forty years old.

Symptoms

- Numbness and tingling in the hands on the front, or palmar, side
- Tingling over the wrist

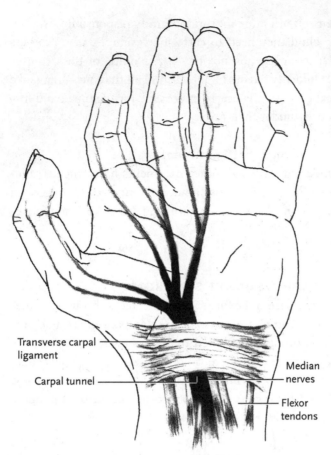

The relationship among the tendons, bones, ligaments, and median nerve of the wrist. In carpal tunnel syndrome, the median nerve is constricted.

Transverse carpal ligament

Carpal tunnel

Median nerves

Flexor tendons

- Decreased sensation in the thumb and fingers

- Pain when holding the wrist in a bent position for a period of time

- Waking up in the middle of the night with numb hands; patients with this problem will often have to shake their hands to regain sensation.

Diagnosis

To diagnose carpal tunnel syndrome, your doctor will look for sensory deficits and for weakness in the muscles controlled by the median nerve. A few simple tests can be done to diagnose carpal tunnel syndrome; two common ones are Tinel's sign and Phalen's sign. The Tinel's sign test is performed by tapping the median nerve along its course in the wrist. If this causes symptoms such as tingling, a pins-and-needles feeling, or an "electric shock" sensation, then you may have carpal tunnel syndrome. The Phalen's sign test is done by pushing the back of your hands together for one minute. This compresses the carpal tunnel, and if it causes the same symptoms experienced with carpal tunnel syndrome, you may have this problem.

An electromyogram, or EMG, is also commonly obtained to definitively diagnose carpal tunnel syndrome; it is used to detect abnormalities in nerve impulse conduction and ensures that the compression is coming from the wrist and not from somewhere more proximal on the arm or neck.

Nonsurgical Treatments

Treatment for carpal tunnel syndrome initially involves conservative therapy; more aggressive and invasive techniques are pursued only if the symptoms are more advanced or if they persist. Initially, you may be advised to take nonsteroidal anti-inflammatory drugs (NSAIDs) and wear a wrist brace, which will help to keep the wrist in a neutral position during the day and especially at night, as we tend to flex our wrists during sleep. The carpal tunnel is at its widest diameter when the wrist is extended, which is why that position exerts less pressure on the nerve.

If conservative measures fail, injection of cortisone into the carpal tunnel can effectively reduce symptoms about 80 percent of the time. Although the benefit may last anywhere from a few days to a year, there is unfortunately no way to know who will benefit most from an injection. Steroids should be injected sparingly and with the understanding that surgery may be required should symptoms keep recurring. The more severe a person's symptoms at the time of diagnosis, the less likely that nonsurgical treatment will be effective.

Surgical Treatments

The most common surgical treatment for carpal tunnel syndrome involves cutting open the sheath (transverse carpal ligament) covering the carpal tunnel; this is called carpal tunnel release. Releasing the sheath effectively drops the pressure surrounding the median nerve, which should allow nerve function to improve. It usually involves an open skin incision (although some surgeons are now performing this surgery endoscopically through a smaller incision), takes about fifteen minutes, and can be per-

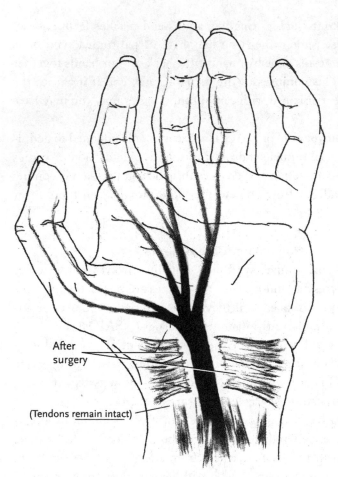

In carpal tunnel surgery, the constricting transverse carpal ligament is released, decompressing the median nerve.

After surgery

(Tendons remain intact)

formed under local, regional, or general anesthesia. Some potential surgical complications include nerve injury, failure to completely decompress the nerve, and pain around the incision.

Patients should expect a gradual reduction in numbness and weakness after successful carpal tunnel surgery. Typically, the more severe the initial symptoms, the longer the recovery time. Some patients may even have residual symptoms.

General Tips for Prevention

Carpal tunnel syndrome is best managed with early diagnosis and treatment. Maintaining your wrist joint in a neutral (not flexed) position helps to decrease the pressure in the carpal tunnel; a wrist brace can thus be used for carpal tunnel prevention. Sports-related carpal tunnel syndrome can be prevented with proper technique and with braces that support the wrist during training and competition.

WRIST ARTHRITIS

Wrist arthritis, as its name implies, is a syndrome involving painful arthritic symptoms like stiffness, tenderness, or swelling in the wrist area.

Causes

Wrist arthritis can occur as a result of

> TRAUMA. Wrist arthritis most commonly occurs when there is a fracture of the wrist involving the cartilage surface of the joint;

> WRIST INSTABILITY. Injuries to the ligaments and bones in the wrist can cause abnormal motion that can lead to arthritis;

> Wear and tear from age-related osteoarthritis;

> Rheumatoid arthritis, which commonly affects the wrists.

Symptoms

People suffering from wrist arthritis will experience its distinctive symptoms of wrist pain, swelling around the joint, and difficulty gripping objects or rotating the wrist (for example, when using a screwdriver).

Diagnosis

Diagnosis of wrist arthritis is made by reviewing a thorough history of the wrist problem and by physical examination. X-ray, CT, or MRI imaging is usually used to confirm the diagnosis.

Nonsurgical Treatments

Managing and alleviating wrist arthritis involves taking a long, hard look at those activities that are causing problems for your wrist. If your job or hobby aggravates your symptoms, you may need to change careers or forgo your favorite pastime. In addition, splints or braces, anti-inflammatory medications, heat, and cortisone injections may help to control your symptoms.

Surgical Treatments

Two surgical options are commonly performed for wrist joint injuries. Wrist fusion involves fusing together the bones of the forearm to the bones

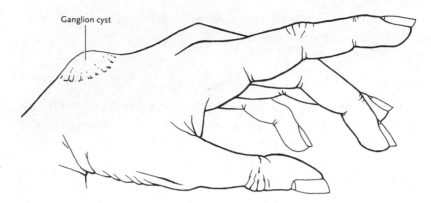

A ganglion cyst is usually a benign bump found on the back (and sometimes front) of the wrist.

in the wrist and hand. Although wrist fusion eliminates all movement at the wrist joint and thus results in some loss of motion, the technique provides pain relief for many chronic arthritis sufferers.

Another procedure, proximal row carpectomy, involves the removal of three small arthritic bones from the wrist—which can provide pain relief while preserving motion. But this procedure is the best option only in certain cases—ask your surgeon whether you are a good candidate for it.

Note that while other joint replacements have become very common (knee, hip, shoulder), wrist replacement is still not routinely performed. Because the results of wrist replacement are more unpredictable, it should be considered only in elderly or rheumatic patients who impose lower demands on their wrists (laborers or young individuals, by contrast, would not be ideal candidates).

WRIST GANGLION CYST

A wrist ganglion cyst is a benign, fluid-filled sac that appears most often on the back of the wrist.

Causes

Wrist ganglion cysts are generally caused by joint capsule damage that results in the synovial fluid "outpouching"—creating a pool of contained fluid outside of the joint space.

Symptoms

The appearance of a fluid-filled bump on the back of the wrist is the classic symptom of a wrist ganglion cyst.

Diagnosis

Your doctor will easily be able to diagnose this condition by examining your wrist.

Nonsurgical Treatments

Although wrist ganglion cysts will sometimes disappear without treatment, they generally grow larger as more synovial fluid is forced into the cyst over time. Indeed, most cysts form a one-way valve so that fluid enters the cyst easily but cannot escape. For this reason, many patients with a ganglion cyst of the wrist will eventually seek treatment either for cosmetic reasons or for pain relief.

The most common nonsurgical remedy is aspiration: inserting a needle into the ganglion cyst and draining the fluid. Unfortunately, recurrence rates for this technique are as high as 50 percent.

Surgical Treatments

The surgical solution, which is usually permanent, involves removing the wrist ganglion and repairing the tear in the joint capsule. This procedure is usually performed under local anesthesia.

BROKEN (FRACTURED) WRIST

Broken wrists are very common injuries in people of all ages. They often occur when people reach out to break a fall.

Symptoms

Broken wrists should be suspected when there is any trauma to the wrist resulting in pain, swelling, deformity, or difficulty moving the wrist.

Diagnosis

In addition to your doctor's examination of the wrist, X-rays are used to both diagnose the fracture and evaluate treatment (an after-surgery X-ray will document whether the bone fragments are in the proper position and are stable).

Treatments

Wrist fractures are often immobilized in a cast or splint, but surgery to repair and reset the bones may be required depending on:

> Whether the fracture involves the dominant or nondominant arm;

> Your age—older patients may not require the wrist strength and dexterity required of younger individuals and therefore may not need to undergo surgery;

> Your general level of activity;

> Any associated medical problems you may have;

> The overall condition of your bones;

> The amount of displacement in the fracture—that is, how far apart the fracture fragments are;

> Whether the fracture extends into the joint space.

Surgery may involve securing the position of the bone fragments by implanting pins through the skin and using a device outside the skin that holds them in place. Alternatively, plates and screws may be used to position the fracture without pins.

JAMMED FINGER

An end-on-end injury to the finger is called a jammed finger. For example, if you catch a pass in basketball against the tip of a finger while it is extended, the ball will drive the finger straight back onto itself, causing a painful compression of the joint. Jammed fingers require immediate attention; icing the finger should begin right after the injury if at all possible.

Causes

Jammed fingers often result from falls or from accidents involving the catching of balls or other objects.

Symptoms

If the injury is mild, you should be able to move your finger with little discomfort only a short time after the injury. If your finger won't move easily or if your pain worsens, however, it is important that you see your doctor.

Diagnosis

Your doctor will likely order an X-ray to determine whether you have fractured your finger. Most jammed fingers will heal completely if there is no fracture or dislocation, although some joint stiffness may linger.

Treatments

Initial treatment involves icing the finger in fifteen- to twenty-minute sessions for two to three days after the injury; later therapy will include the use of heat, passive and active range-of-motion exercises, and techniques to control edema (swelling).

FINGER FRACTURES

A finger fracture, or a breaking of a bone in the finger, can be a very simple problem or a rather complex injury. Anyone who may be suffering from a finger fracture should be seen by a physician immediately to find out how serious the break is.

Symptoms

Some findings suggestive of a broken finger include:

- Pain

- Difficulty moving the finger

- Swelling

- Deformity of the finger

Diagnosis

Your doctor will examine your finger and have you describe details about your injury. He or she should also X-ray the finger and refer you to the appropriate specialist if a fracture is confirmed.

Treatments

A small splint may be all that is necessary to treat some finger fractures; in other cases, the broken finger may be taped to a neighboring finger ("buddy taping") so that the neighboring finger can serve as a splint for the injured one. In more severe cases in which the broken finger is out of position or is deformed, the deformity may need to be corrected, or "reduced," in the doctor's office or emergency room. When external, manual manipulation fails, surgery may be needed to realign and hold the broken fragments in place; in this situation, pins, plates, and screws may be used to secure the broken pieces back together.

TRIGGER FINGER

Despite a popular misconception about the condition, trigger finger does not afflict people who use guns; instead, anyone can suffer from trigger finger, which is so named only because of the position in which the finger is frozen.

Causes

Trigger finger occurs as a result of a change in the relationship between the tendons of the fingers and the sheath that encases them. The palmar (or flexor) tendons run partly through a sheath called the flexor tendon sheath. Although the exact cause of trigger finger is unknown, it generally results from a discrepancy between the size of the tendon and the tendon sheath. In other words, localized inflammation or a nodule on the tendon can cause the tendon to become "stuck" as it passes through the tendon sheath; the result is a trigger finger.

Trigger finger may occur seemingly overnight; for example, you may awaken with the finger locked in a closed position and may have to forcibly unlock it. In other cases patients don't even notice triggering; they will instead complain of swelling at the base of the finger as well as some tenderness.

Diagnosis

Your doctor will suspect trigger finger if you have a finger that intermittently locks in a closed position, particularly if you notice it when you awaken in the morning.

Treatments

Treating trigger finger generally involves taking nonsteroidal anti-inflammatory drugs (NSAIDs) and receiving a cortisone injection into the flexor tendon sheath. If the problem does not resolve with these conservative measures, surgery to release the tendon can be performed. Surgery for trigger finger is a minor, same-day surgery in which the tight portion of the flexor sheath is cut open through a small (less than an inch) incision.

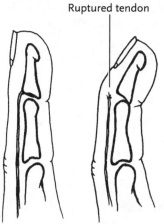

Ruptured tendon

In mallet finger, the tip of the finger is flexed downward (or bent) despite active attempts to straighten it.

MALLET FINGER (BASEBALL FINGER)

A mallet finger is an injury to one of the tendons that helps straighten your finger at the last knuckle joint.

Causes

When the fingertip is "jammed," or forcefully bent down at this last knuckle, the extensor tendon can be torn, resulting in a mallet finger. Although a mallet finger can affect anyone, it usually occurs in athletes who play baseball, football, or basketball.

Symptoms

Patients with mallet finger are unable to straighten the last knuckle of the injured finger, which appears tipped downward.

Diagnosis

A doctor will diagnose mallet finger based on the history of the injury and whether movement of the joint is limited. An X-ray may be done to investigate the condition of the bone where the tendon normally inserts; this image may show a small break or chip off of that bone.

Treatments

Mallet finger is usually treated by splinting the finger for at least six weeks in a special "Stack" splint, which holds the last knuckle joint of the finger straight and allows the torn tendon to heal back into its proper position. Patients may even return to normal activities, including even some sports,

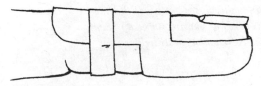

A Stack splint used in the treatment of mallet finger.

while wearing the splint. Although the joint is usually stiff once the splint is removed, flexibility can be regained gradually over time. Mallet fingers rarely require surgery.

FINGER DISLOCATIONS

When the ligaments and joint capsule surrounding a joint become torn, a joint can become dislocated.

Causes

Finger dislocations often result from a fall or an awkward catch during sports.

Symptoms

Symptoms of a joint dislocation include severe pain, tenderness, deformity, and swelling. If you think you may have a dislocated finger, you should seek medical help immediately.

Diagnosis

Your doctor will be able to make a diagnosis based on the appearance of the joint as well as on your description of how the injury happened. An X-ray may also be used to rule out associated fractures or sprains.

Treatments

Treatment of a finger dislocation involves realigning the joint and is sometimes done quite dramatically during a sporting event to one of the players by the team's trainer. Once the joint has been put back into position, the finger is splinted to allow the ligaments and joint capsule to heal. Other initial treatment modalities include ice, elevation, and NSAIDs. An X-ray should be obtained after the splint is placed to ensure that the finger is properly aligned and that there is no associated break in the bone. Wait to start moving your finger until your doctor recommends doing so. Unfortunately, residual swelling and stiffness are typical long-term effects of finger dislocations.

FINGER AND THUMB ARTHRITIS

All age groups are vulnerable to finger joint injuries, which can occur in many athletic and nonathletic activities. Finger joint injuries such as sprains, avulsions (separations), jams, and dislocations can occur in both contact and noncontact sports, including contact sports such as football and wrestling, throwing and catching sports such as baseball and basketball, and sports involving high stress to the hand such as gymnastics. While preventing these injuries is difficult, early recognition and treatment are critical for preventing long-term disability from arthritis. While most finger injuries are mild and resolve with time, others may require aggressive early treatment to ensure good outcomes later.

Causes

Arthritis of the fingers or thumb can occur as a result of inadequately treated traumatic injuries, as well as from systemic diseases such as osteo-arthritis and rheumatoid arthritis.

Symptoms

Symptoms of finger and thumb arthritis generally include joint pain, stiffness, swelling, and loss of motion. These symptoms usually appear gradually and are not precipitated by any specific trauma. Patients with osteoarthritis often develop lumps or nodules around the knuckles of the fingers due to bone spurs (osteophytes); the result is enlarged, swollen, or stiff knuckles. Patients with rheumatoid arthritis, although they often suffer from these same symptoms, can also have more complex deformities of their hands. Patients with rheumatoid arthritis, for example, will often find their fingers shifting away from their thumbs.

Nonsurgical Treatments

Noninvasive treatment of finger and thumb arthritis typically involves:

- Anti-inflammatory medications
- Cortisone injections
- Hand therapy, usually performed by an occupational therapist, in order to maintain motion and prevent stiffening of the joints
- Treatment with ice and heat
- Splinting, which is used to relax and rest the joints (to prevent stiffening in the joint, splinting should be done for only limited periods)

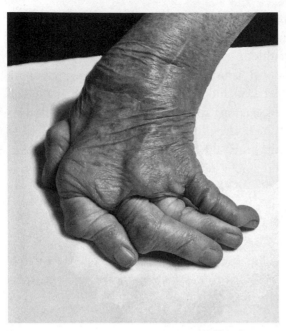

In rheumatoid arthritis, patients can develop gradual deformities of the fingers and knuckles.

Surgical Treatments

If conservative treatments fail, it may be necessary to attempt surgical repair. Possible surgical treatments include removing the bone spurs, fusing the joint, and replacing the joint (although joint replacements are not commonly done because they are not nearly as successful for the finger as they are for the hip, knee, and shoulder).

Exercises for Prevention and Healing

The following simple movements will help reduce joint stiffness, maintain or increase muscle strength, maximize the range of movement in all joints of the hand and wrist, and prevent or correct deformities:

Make a fist (but do not grip tightly); then spread fingers out and repeat.

With your forearm on a table, palm down, turn your hand over until your palm faces upward, then turn it face down again.

Place your forearm on a table or onto the arm of a chair, palm down. While keeping your forearm and wrist on the table or chair arm, lift your hand with fingers straight, then relax by letting your hand drop.

Place your forearm on a table, palm down. Lift each finger in turn as high as possible, keeping your palm on the table, then drop.

Place your forearm on a table, palm up. Keeping your arm and wrist on the table, lift your hand up from the table, then lower it again.

Touch your thumb to the tip of your little finger. Slide your thumb to the base of finger and up again to the tip. Repeat the thumb movement with each finger.

Place your forearm on a table, palm up and the back of your hand flush on the table. Touch the end of your thumb to the base of your little finger and repeat ten to twenty times, stretching out to touch the table between each touch.

Place your forearm on a table with your hand on its side, thumb facing up. Keeping your arm still and, moving from the wrist, bend your hand from side to side.

MAIN POINTS TO REMEMBER

- Some finger injuries require immediate medical attention

- Despite a popular misconception about the condition, anyone can suffer from trigger finger, which is so named only because of the position in which the finger is frozen

- A wrist ganglion cyst is a benign, fluid-filled sac that appears most often on the back of the wrist.

- When the fingertip is "jammed," or forcefully bent down at the last knuckle, the extensor tendon can be torn, resulting in a mallet finger.

- Proper care of traumatic injuries in the hands and wrists can help avoid later arthritis

PART TWO

Treating Joint Pain

Common Medications and How They Work

THIS CHAPTER EXPLAINS MEDICATIONS commonly used to treat joint injury, arthritis, and osteoporosis. From pain relievers to anti-inflammatory drugs to nutritional supplements, this chapter details how these medications work, what their benefits and side effects are, and who should avoid them. There are currently five groups of drugs available for arthritis treatment: nonsteroidal anti-inflammatory drugs, analgesics, corticosteroids, disease-modifying antirheumatic drugs, and biologic response modifiers.

NONSTEROIDAL ANTI-INFLAMMATORY DRUGS

Nonsteroidal anti-inflammatory drugs (NSAIDs) are the most commonly employed weapons against arthritis pain; these drugs reduce inflammation by inhibiting the enzyme cyclooxygenase (which is involved in creating prostaglandins—inflammatory substances that are released in the body in response to trauma and that are responsible for the pain we experience), although they do nothing to slow or alter the degenerative process. Widely used for many forms of arthritis, NSAIDs come in prescription and over-the-counter variations that range from ibuprofen to naproxen, from Anacin to Celebrex.

Aspirin, the best known of the NSAIDs, reduces the body's production of inflammation products that cause swelling, pain, and other

---

The Birth of a New Medication:
From Idea to Drugstore
Enbrel, Remicade, and Celebrex are just a few of the newest
weapons in the fight against arthritis. Yet while they are
flying off the drugstore shelves now, few people know that
it takes an average of fifteen years before a drug is made
available to consumers. Of every five thousand compounds
designed, only one will receive FDA approval and make it to
the drugstore.

---

problems. While aspirin's side effects are similar to other NSAIDs (most
notably, stomach upset), it also inhibits blood clotting and can promote
bleeding.

While all NSAIDs can cause an upset stomach, more selective
NSAIDs, called COX-2 inhibitors (versus inhibitors of both COX-1 and
COX-2, like Advil), are much less likely to produce gastrointestinal side
effects. COX-2 inhibitors were tremendously popular for several years
until concern over cardiovascular side effects (Vioxx) and severe allergic
reactions (Bextra) led the FDA to recall these drugs in 2005. The only one
currently left on the market is Celebrex.

How to Take an NSAID

Taking a drug properly makes all the difference; drug timing, what and
when you eat in relation to the drug, dosing, and many other factors can
mean the difference between feeling better, feeling the same, or feeling
even worse. Follow your physician's instructions (as well as the instructions printed with your medication) closely at all times.

Some NSAIDs should be taken thirty minutes to two hours before
eating, because symptoms will be relieved more quickly this way. Some
of the stronger NSAIDs (indomethacin, phenylbutazone, and meclofena-
mate), however, should always be taken with food to prevent stomach upset.

Like food, antacids may prevent an upset stomach when you're
taking NSAIDs. But both food and some over-the-counter antacids may
interfere with an NSAID's effectiveness. Ask your doctor for the best approach for a particular NSAID.

NSAID tablets and capsules should be washed down with a full glass of water to help prevent the drugs from irritating the delicate lining of the esophagus and stomach. In addition, to let gravity help move the pills along, stand or sit upright for at least fifteen to thirty minutes after each dose.

Finally, remember that these drugs work differently in different patients, so keep in mind that you may have to try several before you find the right one for you. If you're not sure whether your NSAID is helping you, stop taking it for one or two days to assess whether it is making a positive difference in your care.

Symptoms Treated

NSAIDs can help alleviate:

redness, warmth, swelling, stiffness, and joint pain caused by rheumatoid arthritis, osteoarthritis, and other rheumatic conditions;

menstrual cramps;

pain, especially that associated with dental problems, gout, tendinitis, bursitis, and injuries such as sprains and strains.

Most NSAIDs start to relieve pain in about an hour, although relief may not be seen for up to several weeks in patients with severe arthritis. Make sure to check with your doctor about when you should feel relief and how long you should continue your medication.

Side Effects and Risks

While gastrointestinal side effects such as nausea, cramps, indigestion, and diarrhea or constipation are common, NSAIDs can occasionally cause ulcers or bleeding in the stomach or small intestine. Warning signs for these serious side effects include severe cramps, pain, or burning in the stomach or abdomen; diarrhea or black, tarry stools; severe, continuing nausea; heartburn; or indigestion. If you experience any of these side effects, stop taking your medicine immediately and call your doctor. Less common side effects include increased sensitivity to sunlight, nervousness, confusion, headache, and drowsiness.

Other serious but rare reactions are:

Anaphylaxis. The rapid onset of difficulty breathing, swallowing, swelling in the head and neck, and hives may be the result of a more severe allergic reaction. Get yourself to an emergency room at once; on the way, take some Benadryl or inject yourself with an Epi-Pen (epinephrine, available by prescription) to slow the swelling in the interim.

Swelling of the fingers, hands, or feet; weight gain; or decreased or painful urination can be signs of heart or kidney failure. Call your doctor immediately if you experience any of these symptoms.

Precautions and Warnings

NSAIDs should not usually be taken during pregnancy or while breast-feeding.

People age sixty-five and older are more likely to experience side effects of NSAIDs; the side effects also tend to be more severe when alcohol is consumed, because the potential for gastrointestinal complications increases when alcohol and NSAIDs are ingested together.

Taking acetaminophen with NSAIDs can increase the risk of side effects—avoid taking both classes of drugs together if at all possible.

Before surgery or dental work (any procedure that involves a bleeding risk), tell the physician or dentist that you are taking NSAIDs.

Naproxen (Naprosyn)

The NSAID naproxen is used to treat a wide variety of aches and pains associated with rheumatoid arthritis, osteoarthritis, juvenile arthritis, ankylosing spondylitis, tendonitis and bursitis, and gout. It is also widely used to treat mild to moderate pain of unknown origin; while we still don't know exactly how it works, its ability to prevent prostaglandins (inflammatory substances that are released in the body in response to trauma and that are responsible for the pain we experience) from being made probably has something to do with its ability to reduce pain and inflammation.

Ibuprofen (Advil, Motrin)

Ibuprofen is a common fever reducer and pain reliever; like naproxen, it is thought to inhibit prostaglandin production.

Nabumetone (Relafen)

Nabumetone is a common NSAID with a convenient dosing schedule—it is taken only once daily.

Indomethacin (Indocin)

Indomethacin is a powerful NSAID; it has anti-inflammatory, fever-reducing, and pain-relieving (analgesic) abilities. It should be administered with caution to patients with depression, epilepsy, and parkinsonism, because these diseases can become more severe while the drug is being used. Ocular side effects have been noted in some patients who took indomethacin for prolonged periods, so see your doctor or ophthalmologist if you notice any visual changes.

Arthrotec

Arthrotec is a combination of diclofenac and misoprostol. Diclofenac is a powerful NSAID that reduces joint pain, stiffness, inflammation, or swelling caused by rheumatoid arthritis or osteoarthritis, while misoprostol is a man-made prostaglandin that helps protect the stomach lining. Diarrhea and abdominal pain are common side effects, although they typically resolve after the first few days of therapy.

Meloxicam (Mobic)

Meloxicam is taken to relieve the signs and symptoms of osteoarthritis in adults and has similar properties to other NSAIDs. Women who are pregnant or who may become pregnant should definitely not take meloxicam; although it has not been studied in pregnant women, studies in animals show that it can cause birth defects.

Oxaprozin (Daypro)

Oxaprozin, another NSAID, can cause severe sensitivity to sunlight in some of its users, sometimes resulting in severe burns and rashes. Use of a strong sunscreen and avoidance of direct sunlight may be recommended should you develop early symptoms of sunburn.

Celecoxib (Celebrex)

Celecoxib is an NSAID used for arthritis that works by inhibiting prostaglandin production (inflammatory substances released within the body in response to trauma and are responsible for the resulting pain we experience). This drug prevents the enzyme cyclooxygenase-2 from working, and because it does not affect cyclooxygenase-1(which protects the stomach lining) it is easier on the stomach than are other traditional NSAIDs. Celecoxib should not be given to people with a known allergy to sulfa-containing drugs, nor should it be given to pregnant or nursing women.

ANALGESICS

For arthritis pain without inflammation, an analgesic may be helpful. Analgesics fight pain but do nothing to interfere with the inflammation process, making them easier on the stomach than the NSAIDs.

Acetaminophen

The most popular analgesic is acetaminophen, which is recommended as a first-line treatment for arthritis pain. Brand names for acetaminophen-containing analgesics include:

- Tylenol

- Excedrin's "Tension-Headache" formula

- Aspirin-free Excedrin

Prescription drugs that include acetaminophen in combination with an opiate (narcotic) include:

- Vicodin

- Percocet

- Darvocet

- codeine

Although they've been around and used for thousands of years, the role of opiates in pain management is still debated today. While the role of opiates in controlling cancer pain has been well established, their role in the management of noncancer pain is tainted by physicians' fears of patient abuse and addiction. Despite these concerns, more and more physicians are prescribing opiates for chronic musculoskeletal pain as more studies show that the addiction rate is quite low when chronic pain sufferers use opiates appropriately.

Acetaminophen and Propoxyphene Napsylate (Darvocet)

Darvocet is an opiate commonly used to treat mild to moderate pain and is a combination of acetaminophen (Tylenol) and propoxyphene, a centrally acting narcotic (this means that propoxyphene works by changing the way your body feels pain).

Propoxyphene depresses (slows) the central nervous system and therefore should not be taken with alcohol. Because of the potent nature of this medicine, be sure to tell your doctor about any other medicines you are taking, including nonprescription medicines and vitamins.

Acetaminophen and propoxyphene may also cause constipation, so drink plenty of water while taking Darvocet; increasing fiber consumption may also help. Never take more than a total of 4 grams (4000 mg) of acetaminophen a day; many patients take Tylenol with Darvocet, not realizing that both contain acetaminophen.

Acetaminophen and Hydrocodone Bitartrate (Vicodin)

Vicodin is an opiate and antitussive (cough-suppressant) that effectively treats moderate to moderately severe pain. Those who have had a prior allergic reaction to acetaminophen or hydrocodone bitartrate should not take Vicodin, and Vicodin should be used with caution by anyone who has had kidney or liver disease. The use of monoamine oxidase (MAO) inhibitors or tricyclic antidepressants with hydrocodone may increase the effect of either drug, so patients on these drugs should exercise caution.

Tramadol Hydrochloride (Ultram)

Tramadol hydrochloride is a non-narcotic analgesic used to treat chronic pain and pain after surgery. While its action is not completely understood, it appears to bind certain opioid receptors to block pain impulses from reaching the brain. Ultram may cause seizures if used with selective serotonin reuptake inhibitors (SSRI antidepressants), tricyclic antidepressants (TCAs), and other tricyclic compounds (such as cyclobenzaprine), monoamine oxidase (MAO) inhibitors, or opioids.

CORTICOSTEROIDS

Corticosteroids are synthetic versions of natural hormones that your body produces; these steroids (prednisone, hydrocortisone, and methylprednisolone) are powerful anti-inflammatory substances. They also produce side effects that include an increased risk of infection, diabetes, high blood pressure, skin and muscle atrophy, bruising, weight gain, osteoporosis, and glaucoma. Corticosteroids are used to treat rheumatoid arthritis, lupus, polymyositis, and other forms of arthritis; they can be given orally or injected directly into a troublesome joint or a muscle. Joint injections should be limited to about four a year. Because of the side effects mentioned, it's important for patients to be on the lowest effective dose.

Prednisone

Prednisone is a steroid that decreases swelling, redness, itching, and allergic reactions; it is commonly used to treat inflammatory diseases such as severe allergies, asthma, skin disorders, and arthritis. Patients with a history of stomach ulcers or gastrointestinal bleeding should avoid prednisone; it can also wreak havoc on one's emotions, worsening depression in some and leading to emotional instability in others. Prednisone can increase blood pressure and sugar levels, so it should be used very cautiously in patients with high blood pressure or borderline diabetes. Prednisone can also increase the bleeding effects of anticoagulants and cause glaucoma and cataracts.

DISEASE-MODIFYING ANTIRHEUMATIC DRUGS

Disease-modifying antirheumatic drugs (DMARDs) are generally reserved for serious forms of arthritis (diseases like rheumatoid arthritis, psoriatic arthritis, and ankylosing spondylitis) that fail to respond to other medications. Although DMARDs were once used only in the most severe of cases, studies now show that they can delay the long-term damage and joint deformities associated with arthritis. Most rheumatologists today regularly start newly diagnosed arthritis sufferers on DMARDs right away; it is commonly prescribed in a "cocktail" that also includes NSAIDs or steroids. Although most DMARDs are effective, they also have the potential for some very serious side effects. For this reason it is very important to follow up with your physician regularly and follow instructions closely.

Methotrexate

Methotrexate is a DMARD that was first used as a chemotherapy drug to treat cancer; it was incidentally found to have a positive effect on those with arthritis and psoriasis.

The most common side effects include fatigue, nausea, headache, dizziness, diarrhea, mouth sores, increased sensitivity to the sun, loss of appetite, confusion, mood swings, and hair loss. The side effects tend to be most severe shortly after the dose is taken. Taking the methotrexate right before going to bed lessens the impact of some of these side effects on one's quality of life; folic acid supplements can also decrease their severity.

The more serious side effects of methotrexate include liver damage, lung disease, bone marrow failure, and anaphylaxis (life-threatening allergic reaction). Manifestations of these serious side effects may include a dry cough, fever, black stools, unusual bleeding and bruising, yellow skin or eyes, vomiting, rash, swelling, or difficulty breathing.

Because methotrexate can cause miscarriages, women who are pregnant or who suspect they may be pregnant should not take it (pregnancy should be avoided even if the male partner is taking methotrexate). This drug should also be avoided by those with a history of liver disease, and alcohol should not be consumed with methotrexate because doing so increases the potential for liver damage.

Sulfasalazine

Sulfasalazine is another DMARD that was originally used to treat another condition: in this case, inflammatory bowel conditions such as Crohn's disease and ulcerative colitis. Like methotrexate, it was also incidentally found to have a positive effect on reducing the inflammation of arthritis. Exactly how it works is still not known.

Sulfasalazine should be avoided by patients with sulfa allergy, as well as by pregnant or nursing women. Sulfasalazine can also increase sun sensitivity, as well as cause a (reversible) decrease in male sperm count.

Etanercept (Enbrel)

Etanercept is a DMARD and a biologic response modifier (BRM; explained more fully below) designed specifically to treat inflammatory arthritis; it works by binding to a substance called tumor necrosis factor—a key member in the inflammation cascade. Patients who have an infection or who are at risk for infection should not use etanercept. The drug is relatively new, so long-term side effects are not yet known.

Azathioprine Sodium

Azathioprine sodium, another DMARD, was originally used to prevent organ transplant rejection; its ability to improve arthritis symptoms was noted later. Azathioprine sodium use should be avoided by pregnant or nursing women, as well as by men who are trying to conceive. Azathioprine sodium can interact with other medications such as blood thinners, so make sure you tell your doctor what other prescription or over-the-counter medications you are taking.

The most common side effects of azathioprine sodium include fatigue, nausea, diarrhea, loss of appetite, and hair loss. The more serious side effects should be reported immediately—these include pain or difficulty passing urine, unusual bleeding or bruising, swelling of the feet or legs, unusual or sudden weight gain, yellowing of the eyes or skin, and black stools—because the drug can cause certain blood abnormalities and, when used over an extended period, may even increase the risk of developing certain cancers. In addition, patients on azathioprine sodium need to be monitored frequently with blood tests because of the medication's powerful ability to suppress the immune system.

Hydroxychloroquine Sulfate (Plaquenil)

Hydroxychloroquine sulfate was originally used to treat malaria. The side effect profile is similar to that of other DMARDs, with the exception of its potential to worsen psoriasis or cause retinopathy and other vision problems, most of which are reversible upon discontinuation of the drug. Eye examinations are recommended every six months; frequent blood tests should also be performed because of the drug's ability to cause blood abnormalities.

Infliximab (Remicade)

Infliximab, which is both a DMARD and a biologic response modifier (BRM), blocks tumor necrosis factor (TNF) alpha (a substance that can improve the body's natural defense against disease; a type of biologic response modifier) from working.

Preliminary studies have shown that infliximab can actually slow the destruction of joints in rheumatoid arthritis patients. But serious side effects have been reported, such as fever and infection, sinusitis, changes in blood pressure, chest pain, and shortness of breath. Because it is a somewhat new drug, the long-term side effects are still unknown.

Minocycline

An antibiotic mainly used to treat infections, minocycline has provided relief for some arthritis sufferers. Exactly why it works is unknown, although some believe that rheumatoid diseases are in part caused by an infection by the many species of bacteria called mycoplasmas (minocycline treats the mycoplasmas, thus improving the rheumatoid arthritis). Others, however, believe the benefit is merely anti-inflammatory.

Adalimumab (Humira) and Leflunomide (Arava)

Adalimumab and Leflunomide are DMARDs and BRMs designed to block cytokines (key components in the immune system that play a role in certain types of inflammation) involved in the inflammatory pathway. Their side effects can be serious, much like those of other DMARDs and BRMs.

BIOLOGIC RESPONSE MODIFIERS

For those who don't respond to DMARDs, a relatively new class of drugs, called biologic response modifiers, or BRMs, may provide arthritis relief. On the market since 1998, the BRMs help ease severe cases of inflammation by obstructing key components in the immune system. These key components, called cytokines, play a role in the inflammation seen in rheumatoid arthritis, ankylosing spondylitis, and psoriatic arthritis. Enbrel, Humira, and Remicade are three of the BRMs currently approved for treatment of rheumatoid arthritis; they suppress a cytokine called tumor necrosis factor (TNF). A fourth drug, called Kineret, works by blocking a different cytokine, called interleukin-1. The BRMs are injected either into a muscle or directly into a vein and are quite expensive; researchers are still working on less expensive versions that can be taken by mouth.

Possible mild side effects of these new BRMs include redness, pain, swelling, itching, or bruising at the injection entry site, as well as upper respiratory infections. Some BRMs are thought to increase the risk of developing serious lung infections such as tuberculosis or pneumonia, so before prescribing these drugs your physician will need to know if you have any history of these or other respiratory infections.

OTHER MEDICATIONS ADDRESSING JOINT PAIN

In addition to the five categories of most commonly recommended medications, other drugs have been tried in an effort to alleviate the symptoms of those suffering from joint pain.

Gabapentin (Neurontin)

Gabapentin is an anticonvulsant used normally to treat seizures, but it can also treat nerve pain. Exactly how it works is still not known, although it is thought to control chemicals in the brain that send signals to nerves throughout the body.

Antacids decrease the amount of gabapentin absorbed through the stomach, so they should not be taken within two hours of taking the drug. Gabapentin may also increase the effects of other drugs that cause drowsiness, so drinking alcohol and driving or operating heavy machinery should be avoided until you've taken the drug long enough to know your limitations.

Amitriptyline Hydrochloride (Elavil)

Normally used as an antidepressant, amitriptyline hydrochloride can also help promote restful sleep in some patients with arthritis pain. Common side effects include drowsiness, headache, dry mouth, and urinary retention.

Drugs for Treating Osteoporosis

Although there is no cure for osteoporosis, diet, exercise, and certain medications can slow it down. Medications currently approved by the FDA for the treatment and prevention of osteoporosis include bisphosphonates (such as alendronate, ibandronate, and risedronate), calcitonin, estrogens, parathyroid hormone, and raloxifene.

To understand how these medications combat osteoporosis, you will need to become familiar with the bone remodeling process. Bone remodeling consists of two distinct dynamic stages—bone resorption and bone deposition—that occur continuously throughout the human body. During resorption, cells on the bone's surface dissolve bone tissue and create small cavities; during bone formation, these cavities are filled with new bone tissue. Bone resorption and bone formation are usually very balanced; osteoporosis develops when resorption outpaces deposition as we age. Some medications are designed to slow or stop the bone-resorbing part of the cycle without affecting the bone-forming part. As a result, new bone is formed faster than it is broken down (resorbed), so bone density increases slowly over time.

Calcium and Vitamin D

Because calcium is the main building block of bone, eating enough calcium is essential to maintaining healthy and strong bones. Unfortunately, the average American woman consumes less calcium than the recommended amount.

Dairy products such as milk, cheese, and yogurt are excellent sources of calcium because they contain large amounts of this mineral that are easily absorbed by the body. Skim milk products provide as much calcium as whole milk, and they have the added advantage of less fat and

The Calcium Content of Common Foods

Food	Calcium content
Multivitamin	400 mg
Milk (2%, 1%, skim, chocolate)	300 mg
Fortified soy beverage	300 mg
Fortified orange juice	300 mg
Yogurt	295 mg
Lasagna	285 mg
Salmon	240 mg
Taco	221 mg
Cheese	200 mg
Sardines	200 mg
Soybeans	170 mg
Figs	150 mg
Muffin	84 mg
Cottage cheese	80 mg
Ice cream	80 mg
Beans, baked	75 mg
Beans—cooked (kidney, lima)	50 mg
Broccoli	50 mg
Orange	50 mg
Bread	40 mg
Banana	10 mg

cholesterol. Some calcium-fortified orange juices may contain as much calcium as milk (check the labels). Leafy green vegetables also provide calcium, as do fish products, lentils, and beans.

The National Institutes of Health Consensus Conference recommends that the following amounts of calcium be consumed daily (with the total daily intake not to exceed 2,000 mg):

- 800 mg for children ages one to ten

- 1,000 mg for men, premenopausal women, as well as postmenopausal women also taking estrogen

- 1,200 mg for teenagers and young adults

- 1,500 mg for postmenopausal women not taking estrogen

- 1,200–1,500 mg for pregnant women and nursing mothers

Vitamin D helps the intestines absorb calcium; it is found in certain foods and is also produced by the skin when it is exposed to sunlight. Active children and young adults living in sunny areas can produce most of the vitamin D they need from their skin, while the elderly and adults who live in areas less replete with sunlight are at risk for vitamin D deficiency. The National Institutes of Health Consensus Conference recommends the daily consumption of these amounts of vitamin D:

- 200 IU for men and women nineteen to fifty years old

- 400 IU for men and women fifty-one to seventy years old

- 600 IU for men and women seventy-one years and older

Patients already suffering from osteoporosis should take 400 IU of vitamin D twice a day. Taking too much vitamin D, however, can lead to loss of appetite, nausea, vomiting, excessive thirst, and muscle weakness, so intake should never exceed 1,000 IU in one day.

Bisphosphonates

Bisphosphonates are a class of drugs that are used to treat osteoporosis by reducing bone loss and increasing bone density. Side effects for alendronate, ibandronate, and risedronate are uncommon but may include gastrointestinal problems, abdominal or musculoskeletal pain, nausea, heartburn, or irritation of the esophagus. There have been a few reports of osteonecrosis (bone decay) of the jaw and of visual disturbances. Commonly prescribed bisphosphonates include:

ALENDRONATE SODIUM (FOSAMAX). Alendronate is approved for both the prevention and treatment of postmenopausal osteoporosis and has been shown to reduce the risk of wrist, hip, and spine fractures. Alendronate is approved for the treatment of osteoporosis in men and women.

IBANDRONATE SODIUM (BONIVA). Ibandronate is approved for the prevention and treatment of postmenopausal osteoporosis; it is taken as a pill only once a month, and should be taken on the same day each month.

RISEDRONATE SODIUM (ACTONEL). Risedronate is approved for the prevention and treatment of postmenopausal osteoporosis. Like ibandronate sodium, it is taken monthly, on the same day each month.

Calcitonin (Miacalcin, Calcimar, or Fortical)

Calcitonin is a naturally occurring hormone that regulates calcium and bone metabolism. In women who are more than five years beyond menopause, calcitonin is able to slow bone loss and increase spinal bone density. Calcitonin has been shown to decrease the risk of spinal fractures but has not been shown to decrease the risk of other fractures, although many studies are still ongoing. Because calcitonin is a protein and can't be taken by mouth (it would be broken down in the stomach and made ineffective), it is taken as a nasal spray or injection.

While it does not affect other organs or systems in the body, injectable calcitonin may cause an allergic reaction and side effects such as flushing of the face and hands, increased urination, nausea, and a rash. The side effects for nasal calcitonin, although rare, may include nasal irritation and bleeding, backache, and headache.

Hormone Therapies

Several kinds of hormone therapy have been used in an attempt to help ease the symptoms of osteoarthritis. These include:

ESTROGEN. Estrogen alone without progestin (estrogen replacement therapy, or ERT) may be used to treat osteoporosis in women who have gone through menopause and whose uterus has been removed during a hysterectomy. This is because estrogen alone can cause uterine cancer in those patients who still have their uterus.

ESTROGEN AND PROGESTIN. A combination of estrogen and progestin (hormone replacement therapy, or HRT) is sometimes recommended for women with osteoporosis. The addition of progestin cancels out the increased risk of developing uterine cancer due to estrogen. Note that although hormone replacement therapy decreases the risk of hip fracture, it can also lead to small increases in a woman's risk of breast cancer, heart attack, stroke, and blood clots. Consequently, many physicians believe that the risks of hormone replacement outweigh the benefits in most women.

TESTOSTERONE. Testosterone is sometimes given in men to prevent osteoporosis caused by low testosterone levels; however, the use of testosterone to treat osteoporosis has not yet been approved by the FDA.

RALOXIFENE (EVISTA). Raloxifene belongs to a class of drugs called selective estrogen receptor modulators (SERMs), which were created to provide the beneficial effects of estrogens without their potential disadvantages. Raloxifene increases bone mass and effectively cuts the risk of spinal fractures (studies are currently looking at its ability to reduce the risk of other fractures). Potential side effects include hot flashes and blood clots (side effects that are also associated with taking just estrogen).

Significantly, studies now show that taking a bisphosphonate with hormone therapy results in increased bone mass when compared with taking either medication alone.

Bone Forming Medications

Teriparatide, a form of parathyroid hormone marketed under the trade name Fortéo, is approved for the treatment of osteoporosis in postmenopausal women and in men who are at increased risk for fracture; it promotes new bone formation and significantly increases bone density. Teriparatide has been proven to reduce fractures of the hip, spine, foot, ribs, and wrists. It is given as a daily injection and can be used for as long as two years; side effects include nausea, leg cramps, and dizziness.

Glucosamine and Chondroitin Sulfate

Glucosamine and chondroitin sulfate are substances found naturally in the body: glucosamine is an amino sugar thought to play a role in cartilage production and repair, while chondroitin sulfate is part of a large protein molecule (proteoglycan) that lends cartilage its elasticity. Both glucosamine and chondroitin sulfate are extracted from animal tissue and are sold as popular dietary or nutritional supplements worldwide (glucosamine is taken from crab, lobster, or shrimp shells; chondroitin sulfate comes from animal cartilage like shark cartilage).

Past studies have shown that some people with mild to moderate osteoarthritis get as much pain relief from taking glucosamine or chondroitin sulfate as they do when they take NSAIDs such as aspirin and ibuprofen; some other studies have suggested that the supplements may also slow cartilage damage. Recent study results published in the *New England Journal of Medicine*, however, concluded that glucosamine and chondroitin sulfate alone or in combination did not reduce pain effectively in the overall group of patients with osteoarthritis of the knee.

Because dietary supplements are unregulated, the quality and content may vary widely from company to company. We recommend that people interested in taking these supplements choose products sold by large, well-established companies that can be held accountable for the quality of the products they sell. In addition, be sure to consult your doctor before taking these supplements. Recommended doses will cost you about thirty to ninety dollars a month, and most insurance companies will not cover this cost.

The generally recommended doses are 1,500 mg/day of glucosamine and 1,200 mg/day of chondroitin sulfate; a trial period of about six to eight weeks is often suggested. The most common side effect is increased bowel gas.

Children and women who are pregnant or of childbearing age should not take these supplements; in addition, people with diabetes should monitor their blood sugar levels more closely when taking glucosamine because it is an amino sugar that may raise blood sugar levels. If you are taking chondroitin sulfate in addition to a blood-thinning medication like coumadin or aspirin, make sure to check your blood-clotting time more often. Chondroitin sulfate is similar in structure to the blood-thinning drug heparin and has caused bleeding in some people.

The bottom line: At this time, the results of studies investigating glucosamine and chondroitin sulfate have shown that they offer arthritis sufferers mild relief at best.

When to Consider
a Joint Injection

JOINT INJECTIONS ARE DESIGNED TO ease pain and improve range of motion by decreasing inflammation in and around the joint. A relatively new procedure, such injections offer the possibility of better quality of life for those who suffer from significant impairment and discomfort. But as with any medical treatment, not every circumstance and patient are a good match for joint injections. If you are among the many arthritis sufferers who wonder whether a joint injection is right for them, this chapter will give you some of the basic information about the technique, which you might use as a springboard for more meaningful and detailed discussions with your doctor.

JOINT INJECTIONS: AN INTRODUCTION

In a joint or soft tissue injection, a doctor will administer medicine with a needle into a joint (such as your knee) or a soft tissue space (such as the space between a muscle and a bone). Joint injections are usually performed in a physician's office; after your skin is cleaned with alcohol or iodine, a needle attached to a syringe will be used to enter the joint. These shots can be used to diagnose or treat several conditions, including osteoarthritis, rheumatism, tendonitis, carpal tunnel syndrome, and bursitis. The most common medications injected into the joint are steroids and pain medications like lidocaine (similar to the Novocain that your dentist gives you to numb an area in your mouth). Needle aspirations of the joint remove fluid and can be used to diagnose disorders that may be amenable to joint injections.

Common side effects to joint injections include allergic reactions (usually to the medication or to the iodine used to clean the skin). Infections, although serious, are thankfully a rare complication of joint injections and occur at a frequency of less than one in fifteen thousand. "Post-injection flares"—joint swelling and pain a few hours after the injection—occur in about one in every fifty patients but generally resolve on their own in a few days.

The most common reasons that a doctor will decide your condition is unsuitable for a joint injection are infection in or around a joint, or an allergy to one or more of the medications that would have been injected into the joint.

STEROID INJECTIONS

Corticosteroids are a kind of steroid that is both man-made and naturally produced in the body. Because they can drastically decrease inflammation, they are used to treat a wide variety of diseases or problems, especially arthritis. Common corticosteroids include prednisone and prednisolone (both given orally), Solu-Medrol (given intravenously), as well as Celestone, Depo-Medrol, and others (given by injection into soft tissues and joints). One should not confuse these corticosteroids with anabolic steroids, which are used to enhance muscular development and are often abused by athletes.

Corticosteroid injections can be used to treat specific areas of inflammation (local injections); they can also be employed to treat widespread inflammation throughout the body (systemic injections). Conditions that are often treated with local injections include bursitis, tendonitis, osteoarthritis, tennis elbow, golfer's elbow, carpal tunnel syndrome, trigger finger, frozen shoulder, back pain, and joint arthritis. Among conditions commonly treated with systemic corticosteroid injections are severe allergies or allergic reactions (anaphylaxis), asthma, lupus, and rheumatoid arthritis.

Injections of a corticosteroid into a joint can rapidly reduce joint pain and restore function to a joint previously immobilized by inflammation. They can also work wonders in injured professional athletes who need a quick fix in order to bring home the win. But it is crucial to remember that although steroid injections into joints or soft tissues can relieve pain and alleviate inflammation for months or, in a few cases, even years, they cannot cure the underlying problem. For this reason, and because of their potential negative side effects, steroids are generally used only after anti-inflammatory medications and physical therapy have failed.

Areas Most Commonly Treated

The joints most commonly injected with steroids are the knee, shoulder, ankle, elbow, wrist, and thumb, as well as the small joints of the hands and feet. Hip joint injections may require a form of X-ray called fluoroscopy to localize the precise area for steroid placement. Facet joints of the lumbar spine (low back area) may also be injected by experienced rheumatologists, orthopedists, anesthesiologists, radiologists, and physiatrists; these typically require the assistance of radiographic imaging as well.

BURSA. The most commonly inflamed bursa are located in the shoulder (subacromial), hip (greater trochanter), elbow (olecranon), knee (prepatellar), and heel (retrocalcaneal). Bursal injections with steroids can improve pain and inflammation, but it is unsafe to give them when an infection is present.

TENDONS. Some tendon injuries, such as trigger finger or rotator-cuff tendonitis, respond well to corticosteroid injections. Interestingly, some tendons that are inflamed or partially torn can be injected without much risk of rupture (for example, the rotator cuff of the shoulder), whereas others, such as the Achilles tendon, should not be injected due to this rupture risk.

LIGAMENTS. Ligaments of the elbow, knee, and ankle are those most commonly injected with corticosteroids—but to avoid the risk of rupture, the corticosteroids are generally injected around (not into) the ligament.

NERVES. Steroid injections can be used to treat peripheral nerve compression syndromes (for example, carpal tunnel syndrome; tarsal tunnel syndrome, which is similar to carpal tunnel syndrome but occurs in the ankle; Morton's neuroma, in which a mass grows in the foot and narrows the space around the nerves; or herniated disks with nerve compression). About a quarter of patients treated with steroid injections experience long-term or permanent pain relief. It is thought that the steroids work on nerve pain by decreasing the inflammation in the tissue around and within the nerve, effectively decreasing the compression of the nerve that results in pain.

The advantages of steroid injections are that they are easily administered in an office setting, start to work very quickly, and provide more localized effective relief from pain and inflammation than do many oral medications. A joint injection can also help a person avoid some of the systemic side effects such as stomach irritation caused by nonsteroidal anti-inflammatory drugs (NSAIDs).

Side effects of injected steroids are rare but can include depigmentation (a whitening of the skin), local fat atrophy (thinning of the skin) at the injection site, introduction of bacterial infection into the joint, bruising or bleeding around the injection site, and "post-infection flare" (described above). Unique side effects of joint injections involve injury to the joint tissues, particularly with repeated injections. These injuries include thinning of the joint cartilage, tendon/ligament weakening and rupture, and increased inflammation in the joint (arthritis) due to a reaction to the crystallized corticosteroid.

Long-term side effects of repeated corticosteroid injections include weight gain, facial puffiness, high blood pressure, cataract formation, osteoporosis, and, rarely, serious damage to the bones of the large joints. Side effects are more likely to occur with steroid pills than with injections.

Some words of caution: because cortisone can increase blood sugar levels and mask infection, they should be used sparingly in people with diabetes or those who are at risk for infection.

VISCOSUPPLEMENTATION
(INJECTIONS OF HYALURONIC ACID)

Hyaluronic acid is a thick fluid, with a consistency somewhat like an uncooked egg white, that naturally occurs in the synovial fluid of all joints. Hyaluronan, one of the major molecules found in joint fluid, is a major component of hyaluronic acid and is responsible for giving the joint fluid its viscous quality, which helps the joint cartilage surfaces glide smoothly across each other.

When a joint becomes afflicted with arthritis, the amount of hyaluronic acid drops and negatively affects the joint's lubrication. Viscosupplementation involves injecting a series of hyaluronic acid preparations into the knee joint in the hope of restoring this lubrication and relieving pain. Currently, hyaluronic acid injections are approved only for the treatment of osteoarthritis of the knee in patients who have failed to respond to more conservative therapy. Injection into other joints is still being investigated and will likely be approved in the future.

There are currently four FDA-approved hyaluronates (hyaluronan-derived medications):

- Hyalgan

- Synvisc

- Supartz

- Orthovisc

Two preparations of hyaluronic acid are available—a natural product made from rooster combs, and an artificial one made from bacterial cultures. Patients with allergies to eggs or poultry products should not be injected with the natural form of hyaluronic acid. Side effects to injections of hyaluronic acid are minimal but may include mild pain, rash, itching, and bruising at the site of injection; these symptoms usually resolve on their own.

Depending on the product used, three to five shots of hyaluronic acid will be injected into your knee once a week for three to five weeks. Your symptoms may take as long as twelve weeks to improve, and the reason for the delayed reaction is not fully known. In addition to its anti-inflammatory and pain-relieving properties, hyaluronic acid is also thought by some to stimulate the joint to produce more of its own hyaluronic acid.

Unfortunately, viscosupplementation doesn't work for everyone, and every patient's response is unpredictable. Another disadvantage of viscosupplementation is that it has not been proven to reverse or delay osteoarthritis.

Exactly how viscosupplementation improves the arthritic joint is still unclear. Peculiarly enough, while studies have shown that the injected hyaluronic acid remains in the joint only for a few days, patients can experience pain relief for as long as a year. As mentioned earlier, some scientists believe that hyaluronic acid has both anti-inflammatory properties and the ability to stimulate the body's own production of natural hyaluronic acid; however, more research is needed before its exact mechanism of action is determined.

While many studies have recently been performed to assess the effectiveness of viscosupplementation as a viable treatment option for osteoarthritis, long-term studies looking at outcomes and efficacy are lacking. But viscosupplementation injections have been shown to be of some benefit in myriad preliminary studies. From these studies, it appears that patients most likely to experience some benefit from viscosupplementation injections are those between thirty and fifty years of age, with mild to moderate (not severe) arthritis.

POST-INJECTION CARE

Ice should be applied to the injected area for the first twenty-four to forty-eight hours after the injection. If an anesthetic medication such as lidocaine or marcaine (also known as Novocain) was injected in addition to steroids or viscosupplementation, you may experience pain relief as soon as a few hours after your injection. Strenuous activity should be minimized during this early recovery period even if you feel significantly better (because sometimes masking the pain can make you think you can do more than you should). You may also experience numbness if these medications were injected near a nerve that provides sensation, but don't be concerned; feeling should return in a few hours. Now cross your fingers and hope that you are one of those patients who will experience a significant long-term benefit from the injection.

10

Alternative Therapies

ALMOST HALF OF ALL AMERICANS have used at least one kind of alternative medicine in an attempt to ease or cure their medical problems. Of these, baby boomers make up the greatest percentage of patients; those with college degrees and who have incomes greater than $50,000 a year are also more likely than their generational counterparts to embrace alternative medicine. Alternative, holistic, integrative, complementary, unorthodox, and preventative medicines are just a few of the many names used to describe various forms of alternative medicine. Here we define modern Western medicine (that practiced by U.S. physicians) as conventional medicine; these other treatments, which currently encompass a diverse group of medical and health care systems, practices, and products, we will call complementary and alternative medicine (CAM).

Americans' embrace of nontraditional therapies seems to represent a cultural shift. The belief that everything Western medical doctors do is sound while other therapies are ineffective or even quackery has fallen by the wayside; as a society, we have figured out that medical doctors don't have all the answers and that other approaches can help. A surefire sign of the times is that two-thirds of U.S. medical schools now offer at least one course in CAM, which indicates that the American Medical Association and American society are viewing CAM in a more favorable light today than they did in earlier eras. The very presence of a division of the

National Institutes of Health dedicated to complementary and alternative medicine (the National Center for Complementary and Alternative Medicine, or NCCAM) signifies that acupuncture, massage, nutritional healing, herbology, chiropractic, and other therapies have finally gained a measure of popularity and recognition among Americans.

The list of what is considered to be CAM is continually evolving, as therapies that are proven to be both safe and efficacious are adopted into the realm of conventional medicine and new alternative therapies emerge. While the acronym CAM includes both complementary and alternative medicine therapies, the two are different: complementary medicine is used together with conventional medicine (like using aromatherapy to decrease knee pain after surgery), while alternative medicine is used in place of conventional medicine (for example, forgoing traditional high blood pressure treatments in lieu of a garlic diet to cure high blood pressure).

NCCAM classifies CAM therapies into five categories:

1. Alternative medical systems. Alternative medical systems are complete philosophies of healing that often evolved separately and before traditional Western medicine. An example of an alternative medical system in the United States is homeopathic medicine; traditional Chinese medicine is an example of an alternative medical system abroad.

2. Mind-body medicine. Mind-body medicine involves techniques designed to enhance the mind's ability to affect bodily change. Common examples of mind-body techniques are meditation, prayer, and creative therapies such as music or art. Some mind-body techniques that were considered CAM in the past are now well accepted in traditional medicine (patient support groups are one example).

3. Biologically based therapies. Biologically based therapies use as their foundation natural substances such as herbs, foods, and vitamins. Examples include dietary supplements and herbal products. One familiar (though not necessarily sound) biologically based therapy is taking high doses of vitamin C in the hope of preventing cancer.

4. Manipulative and body-based methods. At the heart of manipulative and body-based methods are movements of the body; com-

mon examples include chiropractic medicine and massage therapy.

5. Energy therapies. Energy therapies involve the use of energy fields. Examples include Reiki, qi gong, and Therapeutic Touch. These therapies are intended to affect energy fields that supposedly surround and penetrate the human body.

POPULAR ALTERNATIVE TREATMENTS FOR ARTHRITIS

Some of the most commonly tried alternative treatments for arthritis are:

Acupuncture/acupressure, in which fine needles are inserted through the skin in an attempt to release "energy blockages" and reduce pain throughout the body. Acupressure (called *shiatsu* by the Japanese) is a lot like acupuncture without the needles; the therapist uses his or her fingers, hands, or special tools (wooden rollers, pointers, or balls) to press on the acupuncture points throughout your body to "unblock" your energy flow and restore balance. Acupressure is often considered more a form of massage than a kind of acupuncture, but in actuality it is a combination of both methods. Although there are no authoritative studies that confirm acupressure's effectiveness against arthritis, it does appear to help some sufferers.

Western hands-on medicine, which includes a variety of approaches that range from manipulating the spine or applying pressure to specific points on the soles of the feet; each is based on a unique theory of how pain evolves and is relieved.

Aromatherapy, in which fragrant aromas of "essential oils" are used to try to calm the mind and soothe the body.

Chiropractic realignments of the spine, which are designed to relieve pressure on nerves that may be worsening arthritis pain. Daniel David Palmer introduced chiropractic medicine to the Western world in the late 1800s. According to Palmer, disease was the result of spinal vertebrae exerting pressure on nearby nerves; chiropractic medicine was designed to manipulate the spine and relieve this pressure that was thought to interfere with the healthy functioning of the tissues or organs served by the afflicted nerves and resulted in disease. According to chiropractic theory, manipulating the spine to relieve nerve pressure can restore health and cure disease. Although it isn't clear whether the original theory is correct, it does seem to be true that chiropractic treatment can help acute low back pain; it can also treat certain types of neck and back pain better than Western medicine, massage, or acupuncture can treat them. It may also be beneficial in treating headaches, muscle spasms, knee pain, and shoulder pain. Be careful, however, because manipulating arthritic joints can make them worse (especially if you have associated osteoporosis), you should be sure to consult your physician before seeking chiropractic therapy.

Venom from bee stings to attempt to lessen arthritis pain.

Dimethyl sulfoxide (DMSO), a colorless liquid, used originally as a solvent, that is applied topically in the hope of blocking pain signals.

Herb application. Herbs—roots, stems, or leaves—are applied to the body in an effort to lessen pain, reduce inflammation, or relax muscles, or to provide sedation.

Homeopathy, in which it is believed that "like cures like"—that is, if you show the body what has gone wrong, it can correct itself. For example, if the symptoms of your cold are similar to those produced by mercury poisoning, mercury would be your homeopathic "remedy."

Hydrotherapy, which uses hot or cold water, ice, and steam in an attempt to soothe the body and relieve pain.

Rubbing or kneading the muscles in a massage to try to ease muscular tension and pain.

Reflexology, in which pressure is applied to specific points on the soles of the feet, hopefully to relieve pain in other parts of the body.

Polarity therapy, which is a method of healing based on the concept that life-giving energy permeates every part of the human body. This force is thought to be governed by opposite "poles" of positive and negative electromagnetic energy—hence the therapy's name. When a person's energy becomes misdirected or blocked due to stress, trauma, or other factors, disease is believed to result. Peak health can reportedly be achieved when opposite poles are balanced and the flow of vital energy is uninterrupted. To balance the body's energy, polarity therapy combines various therapeutic techniques from Western and Eastern medicine.

Reiki and touch therapy, in which the "healing energy" of the practitioner is thought to be channeled from the hands of the practitioner to the patient without actually touching.

MORE ABOUT ACUPUNCTURE

Acupuncture has grown in popularity in the United States over the past few decades. According to the 2002 National Health Interview Survey— the largest and most comprehensive survey of CAM—an estimated 8.2 million U.S. adults had tried acupuncture, with more than 2 million using acupuncture within the past year. Today, more than 15 million Americans have used acupuncture to treat diseases ranging from asthma to stomach ulcers, although the vast majority of users seek pain relief. Indeed, many people who suffer from painful diseases such as osteoarthritis and rheumatoid arthritis swear by acupuncture, even if most require several acupuncture sessions before gaining some benefit. Although acupuncture has not been proven to be effective by the scientific community, we do know that it does stimulate the immune and circulatory systems as well as cause the release of the body's natural painkillers (called endorphins).

Acupuncture started in China more than two thousand years ago, making it one of the oldest medical treatments in the world. The term *acupuncture* describes a group of procedures that involve the stimulation of anatomical points on the body. Currently, American acupuncture incorporates medical traditions from China, Japan, Korea, and other countries. The acupuncture technique most commonly used involves placing hair-thin, metallic needles through the skin and manipulating them by hand or by electrical stimulation.

To truly understand acupuncture, one needs to learn a little about traditional Chinese medicine, or TCM. In the TCM system of medicine, the body is seen as a delicate balance of two opposing and intimately related forces: yin and yang. In simple terms, yin represents the cold, slow, or passive principle, while yang represents the hot, excited, or active principle. Among the major assumptions in TCM is that disease is caused by an internal imbalance of yang that blocks the flow of chi (vital energy) along pathways called meridians. The study of acupuncture touts twelve main meridians, eight secondary meridians, and more than two thousand acupuncture points on the human body that connect with them. By stimulating these points, the acupuncturist seeks to remove the obstructions and reestablish the healthy balance of yin and yang throughout the body.

The U.S. Food and Drug Administration (FDA) approved acupuncture needles for use by licensed practitioners in 1996 and required that sterile, hair-thin needles be used. Most patients feel little or no pain as the needles are inserted through the skin, and very few complications have been reported to the FDA despite millions of users every year. Still, complications such as infections and punctured organs can and have occurred due to poor sterilization or improper placement of needles.

The National Institutes of Health Consensus Statement on Acupuncture reports that acupuncture's usefulness has been suggested by many studies, even if these studies have been complicated by poor study design (such as small sample size) and placebo effect. In particular, acupuncture appears to lessen the nausea and vomiting associated with anesthesia or chemotherapy. And an NCCAM-funded study recently showed that acupuncture provides pain relief and improves function for people suffering from knee arthritis.

Unlike many other alternative medicine therapies, acupuncture is more commonly covered by insurance companies. But be sure to check with your insurer before enlisting the help of a therapist; some plans may require preauthorization in order to cover the treatment.

BEFORE CONSIDERING CAM

Because alternative medicine therapies suffer from a lack of standardization (for example, herbs vary greatly in purity and potency), you should take the following first steps in your investigation of any alternative medicine therapy:

- Get an accurate diagnosis from your physician. There are many forms of arthritis, and some are difficult to diagnose (and treat) without standard medical techniques (including imaging tests). While an alternative medicine healer may help your arthritis symptoms, don't count on him or her to make the correct diagnosis.

- Educate yourself about the form of alternative medicine therapy you are considering.

- Ask your alternative medicine therapist for credentials, such as where he or she studied, and whether he or she is licensed or certified by the state or a board.

- Inquire about any possible negative effects of the therapy you are considering, and be very cautious if the answer is "none"—it is unrealistic to expect any therapy to be perfectly safe and effective in all situations and for all people.

- Ask for references, and contact individuals who have been treated for similar ailments.

- Make sure you get good information about the cost of therapy. Remember that most alternative medicine therapies are not covered by your insurance.

BUYER BEWARE

American consumers spend approximately $15 billion a year on alternative medicine therapies, with $2.5 billion spent on herbal medicines alone. While these numbers indicate the public's need and belief in therapies outside the realm of conventional Western medicine, the consumer should realize that alternative treatments generally are unregulated. This lack of regulation means that, in stark contrast to the careful monitoring of traditional medicines by the U.S. Food and Drug Administration (FDA), there is no investigation by the FDA into the safety or true efficacy of these products. Moreover, because herbal supplements are not subject to FDA approval, manufacturers are not required even to disclose the ingredients in these products. So before you try any alternative therapy for your arthritis, discuss your plans with your physician. Some herbal or nutritional supplements have been known to interact dangerously with common medications.

Perhaps most important, remember that although every arthritis sufferer dreams of a miracle pill or magic bullet that can cure this disease, such a cure doesn't yet exist for arthritis—even if some people claim that it does. While most alternative practitioners are honest and sincere, others are more than happy to swindle you out of your money. So safeguard your health and pocketbook by watching for these telltale warning signs:

THE "SECRET FORMULA" TRAPS. Stay away if the arthritis medi-cation you are considering offers no list of ingredients or is based on a "secret formula." Claiming that something is "secret" is a way for swindlers to avoid telling customers the truth—that the ingre-dients are really nothing special.

ONE-STUDY WONDERS. Although a single study can help to estab-lish that a treatment works, try to stick to therapies that several studies have found to be efficacious. An arthritis therapy that may work well for patients selected by one study may not work as well for a different set of patients, so the more studies that find your arthritis therapy helpful, the better. Reputable healers know this, which is why they want to cite as many studies as possible when promoting their therapies. Unscrupulous practitioners, by contrast, may rely only on anecdotal evidence rather than on peer-reviewed scientific literature.

THE CASE-HISTORY GAME. Be cautious of using any therapy that claims its efficacy only through case histories ("Mary Jane from Arkansas swears by this drug!").

CATCH-ALL CURES. Avoid cures that claim to work for all types of arthritis—there is no cure-all. As you now know, there are many forms of arthritis, and all have widely different causes and symp-toms. How could one remedy work for all of them?

THE CONSPIRACY THEORY. Despite some alternative practitioners' claims, there is little incentive for the U.S. government or the aca-demic community to withhold effective treatments from the pub-lic; instead, academic researchers are searching for answers much as you are.

LEGALESE. Shy away from services or therapies that have long, obtuse disclaimers or consent and patient responsibility forms to sign.

Finally, remember to include your medical doctor in your learning process. One of the most difficult tasks we as doctors face is obtaining a complete picture about our patients' health—and patients' embarrassment about considering or trying alternative therapies complicates this task even more. In many cases, we simply don't know what nutritional supplements are being taken by our patients or what alternative therapies are being tried, even if knowing this information could mean the difference between good and great care. Giving your doctor the complete information she or he needs to make a clear diagnosis or treatment recommendation is one of the best steps you can take to improve the flexibility and strength of your joints—and ensure the health of your body overall.

Possible Future Therapies

TO TRULY UNDERSTAND THE treatments in development for arthritis sufferers, it is useful to take a quick look backward, at the discoveries that
have shaped arthritis care until the present day. One of the first advances
was the pain reliever acetylsalicylic acid, or aspirin, which was introduced
by the Bayer Company in Germany in the late 1800s; since then, aspirin
and other medications in its class have been used to treat just about every
type of pain and inflammation. But it wasn't until the late 1970s and early
1980s that we started to understand how aspirin decreases inflammation.
Sir John Vane, an English pharmacologist, discovered that substances
called prostaglandins were released in the body in response to trauma and
were responsible for the pain, swelling, heat, and redness of inflammation.
He then went on to discover the process by which aspirin relieves inflammation; specifically, it blocks the enzyme called cyclooxygenase, which
is involved in creating prostaglandins. (In 1982, Vane received the Nobel
prize for this groundbreaking work.)

Unfortunately, because cyclooxygenases are also responsible for
protecting the stomach lining, aspirin and other NSAIDs—such as the
over-the-counter medicines ibuprofen (Advil, Motrin) and naproxen
(Aleve), as well as more powerful prescription drugs—can cause gastrointestinal side effects such as an upset stomach or, more rarely, a bleeding
ulcer. There are also side effects related to aspirin's ability to reduce co-

The Early History of Arthritis Treatments

Year	Discovery	Application
1872	Salicylates (aspirin)	First drug to relieve pain and inflammation
1948	Rheumatoid factor	Better diagnostic tool for rheumatoid arthritis
1949	Cortisone	Powerful anti-inflammatory medication
1951	Immunosuppressant drugs	Helped decrease the rate of joint destruction in rheumatoid arthritis
1960	Total joint replacement	Surgical procedure to reduce joint pain, correct deformity, and restore or improve movement
1961–62	Identification of uric acid crystals in joints	Made the accurate diagnosis of gout much more feasible
1963–65	Anti-gout drugs	Helped control the frequency of gouty attacks
1963	Newer nonsteroidal anti-inflammatory drugs (NSAIDs)	Improved inflammation management
1968	Link between genes and immune response	Led to a better understanding of how the immune response works in inflammatory diseases
1972–76	Link between specific genes and ankylosing spondylitis, rheumatoid arthritis	Provided important clues to the causes of these diseases
1977	Discovery of Lyme disease	A model for the infectious cause of certain types of arthritis

agulation (the blood's ability to clot); regular users may notice easy bruising or bleeding.

DAWN OF THE MOLECULAR AGE—
AND PRESENT THERAPIES

Because the causes of most forms of arthritis are unknown, most physicians are used to treating symptoms rather than attacking the roots of the problem. But researchers are hoping that improved methods for treating and even preventing arthritis will arrive once we better understand how arthritis arises in the first place. This understanding received a major boost with the dawn of new techniques in the 1980s in the field of molecular biology—the science that studies how molecules in our cells work. In particular, recent advances in molecular biology led to the discovery of two enzymes known as COX enzymes: COX-1, which keeps the stomach, platelets (cells that help prevent excessive bleeding), kidneys, and other tissues working; and COX-2, which is produced when there is trauma and infection. COX-2 is the enzyme responsible for creating the high levels of prostaglandins, which promote joint inflammation in arthritis sufferers. The discovery of two distinct COX enzymes led to specific COX-2 inhibitors that were able to decrease inflammation without as many gastrointestinal side effects; these inhibitors (think of Celebrex and Vioxx) block the COX-2 enzymes, while their predecessors (aspirin, ibuprofen) block both COX-1 and COX-2 enzymes.

Celecoxib (Celebrex), rofecoxib (Vioxx), and valdecoxib (Bextra) were the first COX-2 inhibitors approved by the U.S. Food and Drug Administration (FDA). Although COX-2 inhibitors were touted as great alternatives for patients with higher risks of gastrointestinal side effects, their high cost and concern about other side effects have dampened public enthusiasm and support for these agents. Significantly, two of the COX-2 inhibitors have been pulled from the market because of concerns regarding cardiovascular side effects and allergic reactions—rofecoxib (Vioxx) in September 2004 and valdecoxib (Bextra) on April 7, 2005.

Even as COX-2 inhibitors are coming under scrutiny because of safety concerns, another category of arthritis drugs has emerged as a result of recent advances in biotechnology. The medications, which include adalimumab (Humira), etanercept (Enbrel), and infliximab (Remicade), block tumor necrosis factor (TNF), an inflammation factor critically involved in the body's immune response; consequently, they have been used

Keeping Arthritis Sufferers Employed
Recent studies have looked at what helps keep workers with arthritis on the job rather than at home collecting disability. Factors that seem to influence an arthritis sufferer's decision to quit working include the physical demands of the job, control over work pace or tasks, age, and other medical problems. Future studies should focus on evaluating whether changing job-related factors can help keep workers with arthritis employed.

for both rheumatoid arthritis and more systemic rheumatic disease. Given their relatively recent release, these drugs are most appropriate for patients who have not benefited from more conservative and time-tested therapy. Early clinical tests appear promising; they show that patients treated with TNF blockers may improve more quickly than those treated with older agents. They also suggest that the rate of joint damage is reduced.

TNF is not the only chemical in the inflammation cascade that is targeted by new drugs; anakinra (Kineret) is a newly approved medicine for rheumatoid arthritis that blocks interleukin-1 (IL-1). Whether these inhibitors of TNF and IL-1 will prove to be safe, effective, and affordable in the long term is still unknown. So far, all of the approved forms of these biologic agents for arthritis are available only in an injectable form (into a vein or under the skin); eventually, forms that can be taken by mouth may be developed.

Other exciting but early areas of study seek to restrain as early as possible the body's autoimmune response that triggers arthritis. One approach is a (still-undeveloped) vaccine that would stimulate or suppress certain parts of the immune system; other approaches center on genetics and genetic engineering to predict how an individual might develop the disease and respond to therapy—as well as how that person's genes might be altered as a means of fighting back.

Despite considerable progress and optimism surrounding these newer drugs, we are still faced with the complexities of the body's immune system and the sobering fact that any effort to suppress it makes the patient more vulnerable to infection and other dangerous side effects.

THE FRONTIER: POTENTIAL FUTURE THERAPIES

Newer avenues of research promise even more effective ways of managing arthritis in the future based on known factors that contribute to arthritis development—mainly our own bodies and biology, genetics, and the environment. For example, some arthritis researchers have focused on how the individual parts of our joints work and why they might fail—and have discovered that enzymes called proteases are released early on in osteoarthritis and destroy joint cartilage much faster than it is replaced. Even though everyone has these proteases, some individuals seem to be more at risk than others for this rapid destruction of cartilage. Consequently, medicines that target proteases are likely to be used for treating arthritis in the near future.

Genes play a large role in some forms of arthritis; for example, people with the gene HLA-B27 are much more likely than those without the gene to develop ankylosing spondylitis. Other disease-specific genes have been identified for rheumatoid arthritis, gout, osteoarthritis, psoriatic arthritis, and lupus.

But innate tendencies toward arthritis are not the only contributors to the disease: environmental factors also play an important part. For instance, some forms of autoimmune arthritis, which is stimulated by the body's immune system attacking itself, appear to be triggered by infection. Certain pathogens have already been linked to infectious arthritis (for example, Reiter's syndrome is caused by Lyme disease). Researchers are now looking at how certain viruses such as the HIV virus may trigger other types of arthritis.

Trauma may also lead to arthritis. Several studies indicate that certain recreational or workplace injuries can cause development of the disease, possibly many years later. For example, many soccer players experience twisting injuries of the knee and then are at higher risk of developing osteoarthritis of the knee. Other studies suggest that repetitive movements performed over long periods, such as movements involved in factory or construction work, may cause joint injury. Additional research is needed in both these areas, however, before we can understand how injuries truly contribute to arthritis.

Meanwhile, several new treatments aimed at altering or slowing arthritis have recently been developed. Note that although many show encouraging results, none have yet withstood the test of rigorous scientific study and time.

Cartilage Transplantation

Cartilage transplantation involves replacing damaged or absent cartilage in diseased joints with healthy cartilage (and some underlying bone) from other joints of the body. Although this procedure can be effective in those with very small, specific areas of cartilage damage or missing cartilage (in particular, patients who have suffered isolated cartilage injuries as a result of trauma), it is not effective in patients with generalized osteoarthritis.

Orthobiologics

Metal implants have long been and will likely remain the gold standard for treating and healing musculoskeletal disease. But there has recently been a shift from using purely metallic implants to "repair" disease or fractures to using biologically active implants to "heal" them. The term *orthobiology* refers to the revolutionary practice of using biology and biochemistry to develop bone replacement materials to promote or enhance musculoskeletal healing. Orthobiological products, or orthobiologicals, include resorbable bone and tissue replacement materials.

One example of orthobiologics in action is cartilage replacement/ regeneration, which is also known as autologous chondrocyte implantation (ACI). The technique was initially researched at the Hospital for Joint Diseases in New York and further developed at the University of Gothenburg and Sahlgrënska University Hospital in Sweden. The current procedure involves the use of an arthroscope to take a small biopsy of healthy cartilage from a joint. This sample of healthy knee cartilage is sent to Genzyme Biosurgery's cell processing facility in Cambridge, Massachusetts, where millions of new, patient-specific cartilage cells are grown. A vial containing around twelve million of these cartilage cells is then delivered to the orthopedic surgeon for the second surgery. During this surgery, a small piece of periosteum (the tissue that covers bone) is taken from the patient's lower leg and secured over the cartilage defect. The cultured cartilage cells are then injected underneath the transplanted periosteum, where they will grow and eventually resurface the bone with new cartilage.

While the amount of cartilage replaced is very small, rehabilitation is far from easy. Weight must be kept off the knee for up to six months to give time for the cartilage to incorporate and regenerate. In addition, weeks of physical therapy and rehabilitation are needed to help regain strength; consequently, cartilage transplantation and regeneration are most appropriate for active individuals younger than fifty with localized cartilage defects.

Regenerative Medicine

According to the pioneering biological scientist Richard J. Goss, "If there were no regeneration there could be no life. If everything regenerated there would be no death. All organisms exist between these two extremes. Other things being equal, they tend toward the latter end of the spectrum, never quite achieving immortality because this would be incompatible with reproduction." Indeed, scientists today are trying to find ways not only to prevent and cure musculoskeletal problems, but also to restore the structure and function of damaged tissues. Injured human tissue either regenerates spontaneously or is repaired by fibrosis (scarring); a prominent example of tissue that tends to undergo fibrotic repair after injury is articular cartilage.

William Haseltine, the previous chairman and chief executive officer of Human Genome Sciences in Rockville, Maryland, was among the first to coin the term *regenerative medicine*. Haseltine states that the ultimate goal of regenerative medicine is to define the factors that determine whether regeneration or fibrosis (scarring) will occur after an injury. This knowledge can then be used to design therapies to stimulate the regeneration of damaged human tissues. At its most basic level this regenerative medicine or tissue engineering involves learning how cells interact with various materials (such as scaffolding materials) to recreate healthy and functional tissue.

Haseltine believes that regenerative medicine will evolve in four phases. He describes the first phase as being able to copy the body's own repair mechanisms by mimicking the actions of natural growth factors. Some of the first products of regenerative medicine used for musculoskeletal problems have been these very growth factors. The growth-promoting effects of powdered bone—first observed by Marshall Urist at the University of California, Los Angeles, in 1965—led to the isolation of a family of growth factors called bone morphogenic proteins (BMPs) that, when used surgically, have been shown to successfully stimulate healing of fractures. In recent years, the BMP-related product osteogenic protein-1 (OP-1) has been approved by the FDA and is being used in patients who have fractures that will not heal.

The second phase of regenerative medicine would involve implanting tissues grown outside of the body to restore function (as discussed above in the orthobiologics section). For example, some patients with rotator cuff tendon tears have such poor-quality tissue that repair with the body's remaining tendon is impossible. The hope is that in the future a tendon could be grown in a laboratory that would be able to bridge the defect in the patient's torn rotator cuff. This tendon bridge would have all the same biologic properties of a native tendon but would not promote the formation of scar tissue. To date, in other areas of medicine, several types of bioartificial skin equivalents have been used successfully to treat patients with burns, large wounds, and diabetic ulcers.

The third phase of regenerative medicine would employ technologies that can rejuvenate old tissues by resetting our cells' biological clock, while the fourth and final phase would involve the emerging science of nanotechnology (molecular manufacturing) and materials science. Materials science is an exciting area of regenerative medicine in which novel materials are being engineered to integrate with living tissue without causing rejection. In other words, materials science experts hope to create something that can be placed into the body, fit well in that position, and not attract the attention of the body's natural immune system, which is designed to reject and attack "foreign" materials—that is, materials that are chemically different from the body's own components. The early stages of this technology have been applied to the evolving field of joint replacement, where the key to long-term success is avoiding rejection by the immune system. Researchers have already identified several materials that fit these criteria, including certain minerals and the alloyed metals currently used in joint replacements. In addition, some plasticlike substances that eventually dissolve in the body are currently being used as fasteners in the surgical repair of tissues such as ligaments and tendons.

Therefore, while artificial joint replacement and organ transplantation will continue to be important ways of restoring structure and function, regenerative medicine promises to be one of the biomedical revolutions of this century. The goal is to eventually be able to replace appendages with bioartificial constructs or to guide the repair process along a pathway of regeneration rather than scarring. The advancing cellular and molecular knowledge of the differences between regeneration and scarring, and the success in treating some conditions by gene therapy, bioartificial tissues, and molecular agents, have strengthened our belief that within ten to fifteen years regenerative medicine will have a fundamental role in the medical treatment of musculoskeletal injuries.

A PLAN FOR ACTION:
TOGETHER AND INDIVIDUALLY

Many government and private organizations are working together to best use the nation's resources to both decrease the burden of arthritis for all Americans and increase the quality of life of arthritis sufferers. Called the "National Arthritis Action Plan: A Public Health Strategy," the strategy provides a blueprint to reduce pain, activity limitations, and disability among people with arthritis, as well as to prevent certain forms of arthritis.

But even with a comprehensive plan of action, the task for individuals suffering from joint pain remains daunting. Experience has shown that the full magnitude of potential drug risks does not always surface during the mandatory safety and effectiveness studies conducted before FDA approval is obtained. Moreover, today's arthritis research is so fast paced that the media often report significant new findings before the medical journals can print accurate facts. This method of information gathering often reveals only very preliminary results.

Because arthritis can cause such crippling and extremely painful symptoms and in many cases is difficult to treat, many who suffer from it are willing to take drugs that may produce some relief, even at the risk of significant side effects. As newer medications or alternative treatments hit the shelves, we need to temper our enthusiasm and hope with a critical eye that can judge both their validity and their potentially dangerous side effects. Ask yourself these questions before considering a new arthritis drug or therapy, then consult your physician for further information:

Is there a scientific reason to think the results are valid?

Were large groups of people studied? The more subjects, the more valid the study.

Were the people in the study similar to you in age, sex, race, and arthritis type?

Did the study include a control group (a group that did not receive the new treatment)? If so, how much better did the people who received the new treatment fare in comparison to those who did not receive it?

Have similar results been found by other researchers or institutions?

Has the research been published in a reputable medical journal? If so, which one?

Does the report list any questions that still must be answered before the results can be applied?

Does the report use any qualifying words to describe the findings (such as "some," "may," "preliminary," or "experimental")?

Does the report suggest health actions that people with a specific type of arthritis should take as a result of the research?

Joint pain, whether due to systemic disease or a traumatic injury, is a painful burden for those who experience it. But it will be easier to find the help you need to prevent or treat debilitating joint pain if you educate yourself about how the joints of the body work and how common activities can endanger their integrity—and your health. As we mentioned in the opening pages of this book, osteoarthritis will afflict a great many of us as we grow old. But we don't have to accept this statistic as our certain fate. Exercising, with the aim of both strengthening and increasing the flexibility of the essential muscle groups, maintaining a normal weight, eating enough foods that are rich in calcium and vitamin D, and avoiding activities that strain our joints are all significant steps we can take to help us be strong, limber, and pain-free today and well into our golden years.

Acknowledgments

We would like to thank Julie Carlson and Jean Thomson Black for their valuable editorial advice. Their dedication has helped shape *No More Joint Pain* into a book that is informative, organized, and accurate.

Special thanks also goes out to our wonderful medical illustrator, Stephanie Depalma.

APPENDIX:
Resources for Additional Information

American Academy of Orthopaedic Surgeons
6300 North River Road
Rosemont, Illinois 60018–4262
Phone: (847) 823-7186
www.aaos.org

*While this Web site is directed mainly at educating orthopedic surgeons,
patients may find cutting-edge, accurate information on surgical interventions
targeting joint disease.*

American College of Rheumatology
1800 Century Place, Suite 250
Atlanta, Georgia 30345–4300
Phone: (404) 633-3777
www.rheumatology.org

*This Web site offers mainly information on rheumatologists in your area,
but it also provides accurate and up-to-date patient education materials.*

Arthritis Foundation
P.O. Box 7669
Atlanta, Georgia 30357
Phone: (800) 568-4045
www.arthritis.org

*This Web site offers a broad range of information for the lay arthritis
sufferer, from common symptoms and treatments to the newest developments
in arthritis research. It also provides local information regarding community
events and support groups.*

Centers for Disease Control and Prevention
National Center for Chronic Disease Prevention and Health Promotion
4770 Buford Highway, N.E.
Mail Stop K-45
Atlanta, Georgia 30341–3717
Phone: (800) 311-3435
www.cdc.gov/nccdphp

A great site that offers effective preventative measures against a variety of diseases.

FDA Public Health Advisory
Nonsteroidal Anti-Inflammatory Drug Products
www.fda.gov/cder/drug/advisory/nsaids.htm

Offers information to consumers on the dangers of specific NSAIDs.

Healthy People 2010
www.healthypeople.gov/document

This user-friendly site discusses basic initiatives to help men and women become healthier. Health objectives (many achievable) for the nation to achieve during the first decade of the new century are reviewed in detail.

Internet resources for further information about medications:
www.safemedication.com
www.rxlist.com
www.drugs.com

These Web sites offer important information regarding the indications, risks, and benefits of a variety of medications.

National Institute of Arthritis and Musculoskeletal and Skin Diseases (NIAMS)
1 AMS Circle
Bethesda, Maryland 20892–3675
Phone: (877) 226–4267
www.niams.nih.gov

Ongoing studies evaluating arthritis treatments can be found on this Web site.

National Institutes of Health clinical trials Web site
http://clinicaltrials.gov/ct/show

Users of the Web site can gather information on ongoing clinical trials for a variety of diseases. It is user-friendly and provides good explanations of the risks and benefits of clinical trials in general, as well as information on how to enroll.

GLOSSARY OF FREQUENTLY USED TERMS

acetaminophen (Tylenol)—A nonopiate, nonsalicylate analgesic and antipyretic (fever reducer).

ACL (anterior cruciate ligament)—One of the four major ligaments of the knee, the ACL is the most commonly injured knee ligament. It connects the femur (thigh bone) to the tibia (shin bone).

allograft—Grafting of tissue from a human donor.

arthrogram—A radiographic study in which a dye is injected into the joint before an X-ray is performed.

arthroscopy—Surgery guided by the use of an arthroscope (a fiber-optic viewing instrument), which is inserted through a small opening near the joint.

autograft—Grafting of tissue from one part of the body to another.

BRM (Biologic Response Modifier)—A substance that boosts the body's natural immune system and helps it attack disease or tumor.

CAM—Complementary and alternative medicine. Although the two are related, complementary medicine is used as an adjunct to traditional Western medical therapies, whereas alternative medicine is used as a substitute.

cartilage—A type of connective tissue without blood vessels. It provides a sturdy framework for bone to grow and also coats the ends of bones so that movement can occur smoothly at the joint level.

compound fracture—A broken bone in which a part of the bone has torn through the skin.

CT scan—Computerized axial tomography scan. This imaging technique is used to view slices of a damaged joint in fine detail. CT scans offer better definition of bony structures than do MRI scans.

debridement—The removal of diseased tissue, loose tissue, or bony growths from within the joint.

239

dislocation—A joint injury in which the ends of the bone within the joint are forced out of their normal position.

EMG (electromyogram)—A visual record of how the muscles contract in response to electrical stimulation.

ESWT (extracorporeal shock wave therapy)—During this treatment, sound waves are used to cause tissues to experience "microtrauma," which is thought to initiate a healing response.

fluoroscopy—A radiographic technique that allows one to visualize "live," or real-time, images of patients. It plays an important role in many orthopedic surgeries because it can confirm correct placement of instruments and hardware during these operations.

ibuprofen (Motrin, Advil)—A nonsteroidal anti-inflammatory medication, commonly used to treat fever and pain, especially in patients with rheumatoid arthritis and osteoarthritis.

inversion of the ankle—Trauma in which the foot overextends inward, causing an ankle sprain.

joint—The area where two bones connect for the purpose of movement.

ligament—A tough band of connective tissue that connects bones.

MCL (medial collateral ligament)—The innermost ligament of the knee that connects the femur (thigh bone) to the tibia (shin bone).

meniscus—One of two crescent-shaped cartilages that cushion the knee joint.

MRI—Magnetic resonance imaging. This popular imaging technique can be used to evaluate bones, cartilage, ligaments, and tendons in a three-dimensional manner without the use of radiation. MRI scans provide better soft-tissue definition than do CT scans.

myelogram—An X-ray taken after a special fluid is injected into the spine to offer a clearer, more detailed view of its bones and soft tissues.

NSAIDs (nonsteroidal anti-inflammatory drugs)—This class of medications has become a cornerstone of arthritis therapy. The most common side effects associated with NSAIDs are upset stomach and diarrhea, though these are experienced only infrequently.

open surgery—A traditional type of operation that involves making a significant incision in the body to "open" the area for complete access by the surgeon.

orthotic—A device used to support an injured bone, muscle, ligament, or tendon.

PCL (posterior cruciate ligament)—The most posterior of the knee ligaments, it is located in the back of the knee. Also connects the femur (thigh bone) to the tibia (shin bone).

proprioception—Awareness of one's own body position. Poor proprioception is related to inadequate balance and is a significant cause of joint injury.

RICE therapy—A standard course of noninvasive treatment for most joint injuries that involves rest, ice, compression, and elevation of the joint.

simple fracture—A broken bone that does not protrude through the skin.

sprain—A ligament injury caused by overuse or trauma.

ultrasound or ultrasonography—An imaging technique whereby inaudible, very high frequency sound waves are used to discern the shape and density of various tissues and organs in the body.

REFERENCES

Introduction

Ahmed, M. S., B. Matsumura, and A. Cristian. 2005. Age-related changes in muscles and joints. *Phys Med Rehabil Clin N Am.* 16:19–39.

Aigner, T., J. Rose, J. Martin, and J. Buckwalter. 2004. Aging theories of primary osteoarthritis: From epidemiology to molecular biology. *Rejuvenation Res.* 7:134–145.

Altman, R. D. 1991. Criteria for classification of clinical osteoarthritis. *J Rheumatol Suppl.* 27:10–12.

Altman, R., G. Alarcon, D. Appelrouth, D. Bloch, D. Borenstein, K. Brandt, C. Brown, T. D. Cooke, W. Daniel, D. Feldman, et al. 1991. The American College of Rheumatology criteria for the classification and reporting of osteoarthritis of the hip. *Arthritis Rheum.* 34:505–514.

Andersson, S., B. Nilsson, T. Hessel, M. Saraste, A. Noren, A. Stevens-Andersson, and D. Rydholm. 1989. Degenerative joint disease in ballet dancers. *Clin Orthop Relat Res.* 238:233–236.

Borrelli, J., Jr., and W. M. Ricci. 2004. Acute effects of cartilage impact. *Clin Orthop Relat Res.* 423:33–39.

Buckwalter, J. A. 2003. Sports, joint injury, and posttraumatic osteoarthritis. *J Orthop Sports Phys Ther.* 33:578–588.

Buckwalter, J. A., H. J. Mankin, and A. J. Grodzinsky. 2005. Articular cartilage and osteoarthritis. *Instr Course Lect.* 54:465–480.

Buckwalter, J. A., and J. A. Martin. 2004. Sports and osteoarthritis. *Curr Opin Rheumatol.* 16:634–639.

Burrage, P. S., K. S. Mix, and C. E. Brinckerhoff. 2006. Matrix metalloproteinases: Role in arthritis. *Front Biosci.* 11:529–543.

Centers for Disease Control. 1990. Prevalence of arthritic conditions—United States, 1987. *MMWR Morb Mortal Wkly Rep.* 16:99–102.

Centers for Disease Control and Prevention. 1995. Prevalence and impact of arthritis among women—United States, 1989–1991. *MMWR Morb Mortal Wkly Rep.* 5:329–334.

Centers for Disease Control and Prevention. 1997. Prevalence of leisure-time physical activity among persons with arthritis and other rheumatic conditions—United States, 1990–1991. *MMWR Morb Mortal Wkly Rep.* 9:389–393.

Chen, A. L., S. C. Mears, and R. J. Hawkins. 2005. Orthopaedic care of the aging athlete. *J Am Acad Orthop Surg.* 13:407–416.

Cutolo, M., and R. G. Lahita. 2005. Estrogens and arthritis. *Rheum Dis Clin North Am.* 31:19–27.

Dirschl, D. R., J. L. Marsh, J. A. Buckwalter, R. Gelberman, S. A. Olson, T. D. Brown, and A. Llinias. 2004. Articular fractures. *J Am Acad Orthop Surg.* 12:416–423.

Ene-Stroescu, D., and M. J. Gorbien. 2005. Gouty arthritis: A primer on late-onset gout. *Geriatrics.* 60:24–31.

Falcini, F., and R. Cimaz. 2000. Juvenile rheumatoid arthritis. *Curr Opin Rheumatol.* 12:415–419.

Feinglass, J., C. Lee, R. Durazo-Arvizu, and R. Chang. 2005. Health status, arthritis risk factors, and medical care use among respondents with joint symptoms or physician diagnosed arthritis: Findings from the 2001 Behavioral Risk Factor Surveillance System. *J Rheumatol.* 32:130–136.

Gare, B. A. 1996. Epidemiology of rheumatic disease in children. *Curr Opin Rheumatol.* 8:449–454.

Goronzy, J. J., and C. M. Weyand. 2005. Rheumatoid arthritis. *Immunol Rev.* 204:55–73.

Hootman, J. M., and C. G. Helmick. 2006. Projections of U.S. prevalence of arthritis and associated activity limitations. *Arthritis Rheum.* 54:226–229.

Hootman J. M., J. E. Sniezek, and C. G. Helmick. 2002. Women and arthritis: Burden, impact and prevention programs. *J Womens Health Gend Based Med.* 11:407–416.

Irlenbusch, U., and T. Schaller. 2006. Investigations in generalized osteoarthritis, Part 1: Genetic study of Heberden's nodes. *Osteoarthritis Cartilage.* Jan 25.

Jensen, L. K., S. Mikkelsen, I. P. Loft, W. Eenberg, I. Bergmann, and V. Logager. 2000. Radiographic knee osteoarthritis in floorlayers and carpenters. *Scand J Work Environ Health.* 26:257–262.

Kane, D., and S. Pathare. 2005. Early psoriatic arthritis. *Rheum Dis Clin North Am.* 31:641–657.

Kim, T. H., W. S. Uhm, and R. D. Inman. 2005. Pathogenesis of ankylosing spondylitis and reactive arthritis. *Curr Opin Rheumatol.* 17:400–405.

Kuettner, K. E., and A. A. Cole. 2005. Cartilage degeneration in different human joints. *Osteoarthritis Cartilage.* 13:93–103.

Manadan, A. M., W. Sequeira, and J. A. Block. 2006. The treatment of psoriatic arthritis. *Am J Ther.* 13:72–79.

Mandelbaum, B., and D. Waddell. 2005. Etiology and pathophysiology of osteoarthritis. *Orthopedics.* 28:s207–214.

Mason, T. G., and A. M. Reed. 2005. Update in juvenile rheumatoid arthritis. *Arthritis Rheum.* 15:796–799.

Messier, S. P., D. J. Gutekunst, C. Davis, and P. DeVita. 2005. Weight loss reduces knee-joint loads in overweight and obese older adults with knee osteoarthritis. *Arthritis Rheum.* 52:2026–2032.

Oen, K. 2000. Comparative epidemiology of the rheumatic diseases in children. *Curr Opin Rheumatol.* 12:410–414.

Pearle, A. D., R. F. Warren, and S. A. Rodeo. 2005. Basic science of articular cartilage and osteoarthritis. *Clin Sports Med.* 24:1–12.

Reveille, J. D., and F. C. Arnett. 2005. Spondyloarthritis: Update on pathogenesis and management. *Am J Med.* 118:592–603.

Rindfleisch, J. A., and D. Muller. 2005. Diagnosis and management of rheumatoid arthritis. *Am Fam Physician.* 15:1037–1047.

Sanmarti, R., F. Kanterewicz, M. Pladevall, D. Panella, J. B. Tarradellas, and J. M. Gomez. 1996. Analysis of the association between chondrocalcinosis and osteoarthritis: A community based study. *Ann Rheum Dis.* 55:30–33.

Sarzi-Puttini, P., M. A. Cimmino, R. Scarpa, R. Caporali, F. Parazzini, A. Zaninelli, F. Atzeni, and B. Canesi. 2005. Osteoarthritis: An overview of the disease and its treatment strategies. *Semin Arthritis Rheum.* 35:1–10.

Smith, R. P. 2005. Current diagnosis and treatment of Lyme disease. *Compr Ther.* 31:284–290.

Turesson, C., and E. L. Matteson. 2006. Genetics of rheumatoid arthritis. *Mayo Clin Proc.* 81:94–101.

Tutuncu, Z., and A. Kavanaugh. 2005. Rheumatic disease in the elderly: Rheumatoid arthritis. *Clin Geriatr Med.* 21:513–525.

Ulrich-Vinther, M., M. D. Maloney, E. M. Schwarz, R. Rosier, and R. J. O'Keefe. 2003. Articular cartilage biology. *J Am Acad Orthop Surg.* 11:421–430.

Wedge, J. H., and M. J. Wasylenko. 1979. The natural history of congenital disease of the hip. *J Bone Joint Surg Br.* 61:334–338.

Wojtys, E. M., and D. B. Chan. 2005. Meniscus structure and function. *Instr Course Lect.* 54:323–330.

Xu, L., M. C. Nevitt, Y. Zhang, W. Yu, P. Alibadi, and D. T. Felson.

2003. High prevalence of knee, but not hip or hand, osteoarthritis in Beijing elders: Comparison with data of Caucasian in United States. *Zhonghua Yi Xue Za Zhi.* 25:1206–1209.

Chapter 1. The Back

Anderson, D. G., M. V. Risbud, I. M. Shapiro, A. R. Vaccaro, and T. J. Albert. 2005. Cell-based therapy for disc repair. *Spine J.* 5:297–303.

Assendelft, W. J., S. C. Morton, E. I. Yu, M. J. Suttorp, and P. G. Shekelle. 2003. Spinal manipulative therapy for low back pain: A meta-analysis of effectiveness relative to other therapies. *Ann Intern Med.* 138:871–881.

Baker, R. J., and D. Patel. 2005. Lower back pain in the athlete: Common conditions and treatment. *Prim Care.* 32:201–229.

Bertagnoli, R., J. J. Yue, R. Nanieva, A. Fenk-Mayer, D. S. Husted, R. V. Shah, and J. W. Emerson. 2006. Lumbar total disc arthroplasty in patients older than 60 years of age: A prospective study of the Pro-Disc prosthesis with 2-year minimum follow-up period. *J Neurosurg Spine.* 4:85–90.

Biyani, A., and G. B. Andersson. 2004. Low back pain: Pathophysiology and management. *J Am Acad Orthop Surg.* 12:106–115.

Boachie-Adjei, O., and B. Lonner. 1996. Spinal deformity. *Pediatr Clin North Am.* 43:883–897.

Bono, C. M. 2004. Low-back pain in athletes. *J Bone Joint Surg Am.* 86:382–396.

Botwin, K. P., and R. D. Gruber. 2003. Lumbar spinal stenosis: Anatomy and pathogenesis. *Phys Med Rehabil Clin N Am.* 14:1–15.

Brodke, D. S., and S. M. Ritter. 2005. Nonsurgical management of low back pain and lumbar disk degeneration. *Instr Course Lect.* 54:279–286.

Burton, A. W., L. D. Rhines, and E. Mendel. 2005. Vertebroplasty and kyphoplasty: A comprehensive review. *Neurosurg Focus.* 18:e1.

Burwell, R. G. 2003. Aetiology of idiopathic scoliosis: Current concepts. *Pediatr Rehabil.* 6:137–170.

Carragee E. J. 2005. Clinical practice. Persistent low back pain. *N Engl J Med.* 352:1891–1898.

Castro, F. P., Jr. 2003. Stingers, cervical cord neurapraxia, and stenosis. *Clin Sports Med.* 22:483–492.

Cherkin, D. C., R. A. Deyo, M. Battie, J. Street, and W. Barlow. 1998. A comparison of physical therapy, chiropractic manipulation, and provision of an educational booklet for the treatment of patients with low back pain. *N Engl J Med.* 339:1021–1029.

Cole, M. H., and P. N. Grimshaw. 2003. Low back pain and lifting: A review of epidemiology and aetiology. *Work.* 21:173–184.

De Girolamo, G. 1997. Epidemiology and social costs of low back pain and fibromyalgia. *Clin J Pain.* 7 Suppl 1:1–7.

Eddy, D., J. Congeni, and K. Loud. 2005. A review of spine injuries and return to play. *Clin J Sport Med.* 15:453–458.

Gerr, F., and L. Mani. 2000. Work-related low back pain. *Prim Care.* 27:865–876.

Gerszten, P. C., W. C. Welch, and J. T. King, Jr. 2006. Quality of life assessment in patients undergoing nucleoplasty-based percutaneous discectomy. *J Neurosurg Spine.* 4:36–42.

Harte, A. A., G. D. Baxter, and J. H. Gracey. 2003. The efficacy of traction for back pain: A systematic review of randomized controlled trials. *Arch Phys Med Rehabil.* 84:1542–1553.

Hurwitz, E. L., H. Morgenstern, G. F. Kominski, F. Yu, and L. M. Chiang. 2006. A randomized trial of chiropractic and medical care for patients with low back pain: Eighteen-month follow-up outcomes from the UCLA low back pain study. *Spine.* 31:611–621.

Jordon, J., T. Shawver Morgan, and J. Weinstein. 2005. Herniated lumbar disc. *Clin Evid.* 13:1445–1458.

Khadilkar, A., S. Milne, L. Brosseau, G. Wells, P. Tugwell, V. Robinson, B. Shea, and M. Saginur. 2005. Transcutaneous electrical nerve stimulation for the treatment of chronic low back pain: A systematic review. *Spine.* 30:2657–2666.

Lenssinck, M. L., A. C. Frijlink, M. Y. Berger, S. M. Bierman-Zeinstra, K. Verkerk, and A. P. Verhagen. 2005. Effect of bracing and other conservative interventions in the treatment of idiopathic scoliosis in adolescents: A systematic review of clinical trials. *Phys Ther.* 85:1329–1339.

Manheimer, E., A. White, B. Berman, K. Forys, and E. Ernst. 2005. Meta-analysis: Acupuncture for low back pain. *Ann Intern Med.* 142:651–663.

Maroon, J. C. 2002. Current concepts in minimally invasive discectomy. *Neurosurgery.* 51:137–145.

Muto, M., C. Andreula, and M. Leonardi. 2004. Treatment of herniated lumbar disc by intradiscal and intraforaminal oxygen-ozone (O2-O3) injection. *J Neuroradiol.* 31:183–189.

Parent, S., P. O. Newton, and D. R. Wenger. 2005. Adolescent idiopathic scoliosis: Etiology, anatomy, natural history, and bracing. *Instr Course Lect.* 54:529–536.

Petersen, T., P. Kryger, C. Ekdahl, S. Olsen, and S. Jacobsen. 2002. The effect of McKenzie therapy as compared with that of intensive strengthening training for the treatment of patients with subacute or chronic low back pain: A randomized controlled trial. *Spine.* 27:1702–1709.

Reamy, B. V., and J. B. Slakey. 2001. Adolescent idiopathic scoliosis: Review and current concepts. *Am Fam Physician.* 64:111–116.

Sengupta, D. K., and H. N. Herkowitz. 2003. Lumbar spinal stenosis: Treatment strategies and indications for surgery. *Orthop Clin North Am.* 34:281–295.

Szpalski, M., and R. Gunzburg. 2003. Lumbar spinal stenosis in the elderly: An overview. *Eur Spine J.* 12 (suppl): 70–175.

Truumees, E. 2005. Spinal stenosis: Pathophysiology, clinical and radiologic classification. *Instr Course Lect.* 54:287–302.

Truumees, E., and H. N. Herkowitz. 2001. Lumbar spinal stenosis: Treatment options. *Instr Course Lect.* 50:153–161.

Vaccaro, A. R., D. H. Kim, D. S. Brodke, M. Harris, J. R. Chapman, T. Schildhauer, M. L. Routt, and R. C. Sasso. 2004. Diagnosis and management of thoracolumbar spine fractures. *Instr Course Lect.* 53:359–373.

Van Tulder, M., and B. Koes. 2004. Low back pain (chronic). *Clin Evid.* 12:1659–1684.

———. 2004. Low back pain (acute). *Clin Evid.* 12:1643–1658.

Yuan, P. S., R. E. Booth, Jr., and T. J. Albert. 2005. Nonsurgical and surgical management of lumbar spinal stenosis. *Instr Course Lect.* 54:303–312.

Chapter 2. The Hip

Abboud, J. A., R. V. Patel, R. E. Booth, Jr., and D. G. Nazarian. 2004. Outcomes of total hip arthroplasty are similar for patients with displaced femoral neck fractures and osteoarthritis. *Clin Orthop Relat Res.* 421:151–154.

Anderson, K., S. M. Strickland, and R. Warren. 2001. Hip and groin injuries in athletes. *Am J Sports Med.* 29:521–533.

Asada, T. 2005. Role of psychiatry in prevention of accidental falling in the aged. *Seishin Shinkeigaku Zasshi.* 107:378–382.

Beer, C., and E. Giles. 2005. Hip fracture: Challenges in prevention and management. *Aust Fam Physician.* 34:673–676.

Butcher, J. D., K. L. Salzman, and W. A. Lillegard. 1996. Lower extremity bursitis. *Am Fam Physician.* 53:2317–2324.

Clanton, T. O., and K. J. Coupe. 1998. Hamstring strains in athletes: Diagnosis and treatment. *J Am Acad Orthop Surg.* 6:237–248.

Compston, J. 2001. Secondary causes of osteoporosis in men. *Calcif Tissue Int.* 69:193–195.

Cosman, F., J. Nieves, L. Komar, G. Ferrer, J. Herbert, C. Formica, V. Shen, and R. Lindsay. 1998. Fracture history and bone loss in patients with MS. *Neurology.* 51:1161–1165.

Croisier, J. L. 2004. Factors associated with recurrent hamstring injuries. *Sports Med.* 34:681–695.

Cummings, S. R., M. C. Nevitt, W. S. Browner, K. Stone, K. M. Fox, K. E. Ensrud, J. Cauley, D. Black, and T. M. Vogt. 1995. Risk factors for hip fracture in white women: Study of Osteoporotic Fractures Research Group. *N Engl J Med.* 332:767–773.

DiGioia, A. M., III, S. Blendea, B. Jaramaz, and T. J. Levison. 2004. Less invasive total hip arthroplasty using navigational tools. *Instr Course Lect.* 53:157–164.

Drezner, J. A. 2003. Practical management: Hamstring muscle injuries. *Clin J Sport Med.* 13:48–52.

Farrell, C. M., B. D. Springer, G. J. Haidukewych, and B. F. Morrey. 2005. Motor nerve palsy following primary total hip arthroplasty. *J Bone Joint Surg Am.* 87:2619–2625.

Felson, D. T. 2005. Relation of obesity and of vocational and avocational risk factors to osteoarthritis. *J Rheumatol.* 32:1133–1135.

Genever, R. W., T. W. Downes, and P. Medcalf. 2005. Fracture rates in Parkinson's disease compared with age- and gender-matched controls: A retrospective cohort study. *Ageing.* 34:21–24.

Gross, A. F., S. Fickert, and K. P. Gunther. 2005. Obesity and arthritis. *Orthopade.* 34:638–644.

Holmich, P., P. Uhrskou, L. Ulnits, I. L. Kanstrup, M. B. Nielsen, A. M. Bjerg, and K. Krogsgaard. 1999. Effectiveness of active physi-

cal training as treatment for long-standing adductor-related groin
pain in athletes: Randomised trial. *Lancet* 353:439–443.

Huo, M. H., and N. F. Gilbert. 2005. What's new in hip arthroplasty.
J Bone Joint Surg Am. 87:2133–2146.

Jacqmin-Gadda, H., A. Fourrier, D. Commenges, and J. F. Dartigues.
1998. Risk factors for fractures in the elderly. *Epidemiology.* 9:417–
423.

Kannus, P., J. Parkkari, S. Niemi, M. Pasanen, M. Palvanen,
M. Jarvinen, and I. Vuori. 2000. Prevention of hip fracture in elderly
people with use of a hip protector. *N Engl J Med.* 343:1506–1513.

Kaplan, F. S., M. Pertschuk, M. Fallon, and J. Haddad. 1986. Osteoporosis and hip fracture in a young woman with anorexia nervosa.
Clin Orthop Relat Res. 212:250–254.

Karlsson, M. K., P. Gerdhem, and H. G. Ahlborg. 2005. The prevention
of osteoporotic fractures. *J Bone Joint Surg Br.* 87:1320–1327.

Kaz Kaz, H., D. Johnson, S. Kerry, U. Chinappen, K. Tweed, and
S. Patel. 2004. Fall-related risk factors and osteoporosis in women
with rheumatoid arthritis. *Rheumatology.* 43:1267–1271.

Kirk, J. K., M. Nichols, and J. G. Spangler. 2002. Use of a peripheral
dexa measurement for osteoporosis screening. *Fam Med.* 34:201–205.

Kujala, U. M., S. Orava, and M. Jarvinen. 1997. Hamstring injuries:
Current trends in treatment and prevention. *Sports Med.* 23:397–
404.

Lieberman, J. R., P. S. Romano, G. Mahendra, J. Keyzer, and M. Chil-
cott. 2006. The treatment of hip fractures: Variations in care. *Clin
Orthop Relat Res.* 442:239–244.

Lin, J. T., and J. M. Lane. 2004. Prevention of hip fractures: Medical
and nonmedical management. *Instr Course Lect.* 53:417–425.

Lu-Yao, G. L., J. A. Baron, J. A. Barrett, and E. S. Fisher. 1994. Treatment and survival among elderly Americans with hip fractures: A
population-based study. *Am J Public Health.* 84:1287–1291.

Lynch, S. A., and P. A. Renstrom. 1999. Groin injuries in sport: Treatment strategies. *Sports Med.* 28:137–144.

Maloney, W. J., and J. A. Keeney. 2004. Leg length discrepancy after
total hip arthroplasty. *J Arthroplasty.* 19:108–110.

McAlindon, T. E., M. P. LaValley, J. P. Gulin, and D. T. Felson. 2000.
Glucosamine and chondroitin for treatment of osteoarthritis: A
systematic quality assessment and meta-analysis. *JAMA.* 283:1469–
1475.

Misra, M., G. I. Papakostas, and A. Klibanski. 2004. Effects of psychiatric disorders and psychotropic medications on prolactin and bone metabolism. *J Clin Psychiatry*. 65:1607–1618.

Nicholas, S. J., and T. F. Tyler. 2002. Adductor muscle strains in sport. *Sports Med*. 32:339–344.

Ogonda, L., R. Wilson, P. Archbold, M. Lawlor, P. Humphreys, S. O'Brien, and D. Beverland. 2004. A minimal-incision technique in total hip arthroplasty does not improve early postoperative outcomes: A prospective, randomized, controlled trial. *J Bone Joint Surg Am*. 87:701–710.

Orchard, J., T. M. Best, and G. M. Verrall. 2005. Return to play following muscle strains. *Clin J Sport Med*. 15:436–441.

Pagnano, M. W., J. Leone, D. G. Lewallen, and A. D. Hanssen. 2005. Two-incision THA had modest outcomes and some substantial complications. *Clin Orthop Relat Res*. 441:86–90.

Reginster, J. Y., and N. Sarlet. 2006. The treatment of severe postmenopausal osteoporosis: A review of current and emerging therapeutic options. *Treat Endocrinol*. 5:15–23.

Rupp, J. D., and L. W. Schneider. 2004. Injuries to the hip joint in frontal motor-vehicle crashes: biomechanical and real-world perspectives. *Orthop Clin North Am*. 35: 493–504.

Schiff, R. L., S. R. Kahn, I. Shrier, C. Strulovitch, W. Hammouda, E. Cohen, and D. Zukor. 2005. Identifying orthopedic patients at high risk for venous thromboembolism despite thromboprophylaxis. *Chest*. 128:3364–3371.

Shbeeb, M. I., and E. L. Matteson. 1996. Trochanteric bursitis (greater trochanter pain syndrome). *Mayo Clin Proc*. 71:565–569.

Snider, R. K. 1997. Trochanteric bursitis. In *Essentials of Musculoskeletal Care*. Rosemont, Ill.: American Academy of Orthopaedic Surgeons.

Souverein, P. C., D. J. Webb, H. Petri, J. Weil, T. P. Van Staa, and T. Egberts. 2005. Incidence of fractures among epilepsy patients: A population-based retrospective cohort study in the General Practice Research Database. *Epilepsia*. 46:304–310.

Stevens J. A., and S. Olson. 2000. Reducing falls and resulting hip fractures among older women. *MMWR Recomm Rep*. 49:3–12.

Stove, J. 2005. Conservative therapy of arthritis. *Orthopade*. 34:613–621.

Tak, E., P. Staats, A. Van Hespen, and M. Hopman-Rock. 2005. The effects of an exercise program for older adults with osteoarthritis of the hip. *J Rheumatol*. 32:1106–1113.

Van der Esch, M., M. Heijmans, and J. Dekker. 2003. Factors contributing to possession and use of walking aids among persons with rheumatoid arthritis and osteoarthritis. *Arthritis Rheum.* 49:838–842.

Vestergaard, P., and L. Mosekilde. 2003. Hyperthyroidism, bone mineral, and fracture risk: A meta-analysis. *Thyroid.* 13:585–593.

Weisman, S. M. 2005. The calcium connection to bone health across a woman's lifespan: A roundtable. *J Reprod Med.* 50:879–884.

Wilkins, C. H., and S. J. Birge. 2005. Prevention of osteoporotic fractures in the elderly. *Am J Med.* 118:1190–1195.

Worrell, T. W. 1994. Factors associated with hamstring injuries: An approach to treatment and preventative measures. *Sports Med.* 17:338–345.

Zuckerman, J. D. 1996. Hip fracture. *N Engl J Med.* 334:1519–1525.

Chapter 3. The Knee

Ahmad, C. S., A. M. Clark, N. Heilmann, J. S. Schoeb, T. R. Gardner, and W. N. Levine. 2005. Effect of gender and maturity on quadriceps-to-hamstring strength ratio and anterior cruciate ligament laxity. *Am J Sports Med.* Oct. 6.

Albright J. P., A. Saterbak, and J. Stokes. 1995. Use of knee braces in sport: Current recommendations. *Sports Med.* 20:281–301.

Aminaka, N., and P. A. Gribble. 2005. A systematic review of the effects of therapeutic taping on patellofemoral pain syndrome. *J Athl Train.* 40:341–351.

Arnoczky, S. P., and R. F. Warren. 1983. The microvasculature of the meniscus and its response to injury: An experimental study in the dog. *Am J Sports Med.* 11:131–141.

Bach, B. R., Jr., M. Dennis, J. Balin, and J. Hayden. 2005. Arthroscopic meniscal repair: Analysis of treatment failures. *J Knee Surg.* 18:278–284.

Baquie, P. 2002. Lower limb taping. *Aust Fam Physician.* 31:451–452.

Baratz, M. E., F. H. Fu, and R. Mengato. 1986. Meniscal tears: The effect of meniscectomy and of repair on intraarticular contact areas and stress in the human knee. A preliminary report. *Am J Sports Med.* 14:270–275.

Blazina, M. E., R. K. Kerlan, F. W. Jobe, V. S. Carter, and G. J. Carlson. 1973. Jumper's knee. *Orthop Clin North Am.* 4:665–678.

Caraffa, A., G. Cerulli, M. Projetti, G. Aisa, and A. Rizzo. 1996. Prevention of anterior cruciate ligament injuries in soccer: A prospective controlled study of proprioceptive training. *Knee Surg Sports Traumatol Arthrosc.* 4:19–21.

Colosimo, A. J., and F. H. Bassett III. 1990. Jumper's knee: Diagnosis and treatment. *Orthop Rev.* 19:139–149.

Dowd, G. S. 2004. Reconstruction of the posterior cruciate ligament: Indications and results. *J Bone Joint Surg Br.* 86:480–491.

Dugan, S. A. 2005. Sports-related knee injuries in female athletes: What gives? *Am J Phys Med Rehabil.* 84:122–130.

Felson, D. T. 2004. Risk factors for osteoarthritis: Understanding joint vulnerability. *Clin Orthop Relat Res.* 427:16–21.

Forster, M. C. 2003. Survival analysis of primary cemented total knee arthroplasty: Which designs last. *J Arthroplasty.* 18:265–270.

Fritz, R. C. 2003. MR imaging of meniscal and cruciate ligament injuries. *Magn Reson Imaging Clin N Am.* 11:283–293.

Griffin, L. Y., J. Agel, M. J. Albohm, E. A. Arendt, R. W. Dick, W. E. Garrett, J. G. Garrick, et al. 2000. Noncontact anterior cruciate ligament injuries: Risk factors and prevention strategies. *J Am Acad Orthop Surg.* 8:141–150.

Kannus, P. 1988. Long-term results of conservatively treated medial collateral ligament injuries of the knee joint. *Clin Orthop Relat Res.* 226:103–112.

Kotsovolos, E. S., M. E. Hantes, D. S. Mastrokalos, O. Lorbach, and H. H. Paessler. 2006. Results of all-inside meniscal repair with the FasT-Fix meniscal repair system. *Arthroscopy.* 22:3–9.

Loughlin, J. 2005. Polymorphism in signal transduction is a major route through which osteoarthritis susceptibility is acting. *Curr Opin Rheumatol.* 17:629–633.

Lun, V. M., J. P. Wiley, W. H. Meeuwisse, and T. L. Yanagawa. 2005. Effectiveness of patellar bracing for treatment of patellofemoral pain syndrome. *Clin J Sport Med.* 15:235–240.

Manninen, P., H. Riihimaki, M. Heliovaara, and O. Suomalainen. 2004. Weight changes and the risk of knee osteoarthritis requiring arthroplasty. *Ann Rheum Dis.* 63:1434–1437.

Margheritini, F., and P. P. Mariani. 2003. Diagnostic evaluation of posterior cruciate ligament injuries. *Knee Surg Sports Traumatol Arthrosc.* 11:282–288.

Markey, K. L. 1991. Functional rehabilitation of the cruciate-deficient knee. *Sports Med.* 12:407–417.

Matava, M. J. 1996. Patellar tendon ruptures. *J Am Acad Orthop Surg.* 4:287–296.

Miller, M. D., D. E. Cooper, G. C. Fanelli, C. D. Harner, and R. F. LaPrade. 2002. Posterior cruciate ligament: Current concepts. *Instr Course Lect.* 51:347–351.

Millet, C., and D. Drez, Jr. 1987. Knee Braces. *Orthopedics.* 10:1777–1780.

Pagnano, M. W., H. D. Clarke, D. J. Jacofsky, A. Amendola, and J. A. Repicci. 2005. Surgical treatment of the middle-aged patient with arthritic knees. *Instr Course Lect.* 54:251–259.

Post, W. R. 2005. Patellofemoral pain: Results of nonoperative treatment. *Clin Orthop Relat Res.* 436:55–59.

Reider, B. 1996. Medial collateral ligament injuries in athletes. *Sports Med.* 21:147–156.

Smith, A. J., J. Gidley, J. R. Sandy, M. J. Perry, C. J. Elson, J. R. Kirwan, T. D. Spector, M. Doherty, J. L. Bidwell, and J. P. Mansell. 2005. Haplotypes of the low-density lipoprotein receptor-related protein 5 (LRP5) gene: Are they a risk factor in osteoarthritis? *Osteoarthritis Cartilage.* 13:608–613.

Warden, S. J., and P. Brukner. 2003. Patellar tendinopathy. *Clin Sports Med.* 22:743–759.

Watanabe, H., S. Akizuki, and T. Takizawa. 2004. Survival analysis of a cementless, cruciate-retaining total knee arthroplasty: Clinical and radiographic assessment 10 to 13 years after surgery. *J Bone Joint Surg Br.* 86:824–829.

Wilson, J. J., and T. M. Best. 2005. Common overuse tendon problems: A review and recommendations for treatment. *Am Fam Physician.* 72:811–818.

Wind, W. M., Jr., J. A. Bergfeld, and R. D. Parker. Evaluation and treatment of posterior cruciate ligament injuries: Revisited. 2004. *Am J Sports Med.* 32:1765–1775.

Chapter 4. The Foot and Ankle

Baker, C. L., and J. M. Graham, Jr. 1993. Current concepts in ankle arthroscopy. *Orthopedics.* 16:1027–1035.

Beynnon, B. D., D. F. Murphy, and D. M. Alosa. 2002. Predictive factors for lateral ankle sprains: A literature review. *J Athl Train.* 37:376–380.

Brosky, T., J. Nyland, A. Nitz, and D. N. Caborn. 1995. The ankle ligaments: Consideration of syndesmotic injury and implications for rehabilitation. *J Orthop Sports Phys Ther.* 21:197–205.

Buchbinder, R. 2004. Clinical practice: Plantar fasciitis. *N Engl J Med.* 350:2159–2166.

Calder, J. D., and T. S. Saxby. 2003. Surgical treatment of insertional Achilles tendinosis. *Foot Ankle Int.* 24:119–121.

Clanton, T. O., and J. J. Ford. 1994. Turf toe injury. *Clin Sports Med.* 13:731–741.

Clanton, T. O., and P. Paul. 2002. Syndesmosis injuries in athletes. *Foot Ankle Clin.* 7:529–549.

Cohen R. S., and T. A. Balcom. 2003. Current treatment options for ankle injuries: Lateral ankle sprain, Achilles tendonitis, and Achilles rupture. *Curr Sports Med Rep.* 2:251–254.

Cole, C., C. Seto, and J. Gazewood. 2005. Plantar fasciitis: Evidence-based review of diagnosis and therapy. *Am Fam Physician.* 72:2237–2242.

Coughlin, M. J., and P. S. Shurnas. 2004. Hallux rigidus. *J Bone Joint Surg Am.* 86:119–130.

Cullen, N. P., and D. Singh. 2006. Plantar fasciitis: A review. *Br J Hosp Med* (Lond). 67:72–76.

Dyck, D. D., Jr., and L. A. Boyajian-O'Neill. 2004. Plantar fasciitis. *Clin J Sport Med.* 14:305–309.

Frey, C. 2001. Ankle Sprains. *Instr Course Lect.* 50:515–520.

Gehrmann, R. M., S. Rajan, D. V. Patel, and C. Bibbo. 2005. Athletes' ankle injuries: Diagnosis and management. *Am J Orthop.* 34:551–561.

Gross, M. T., and H. Y. Liu. 2003. The role of ankle bracing for prevention of ankle sprain injuries. *J Orthop Sports Phys Ther.* 33:572–577.

Hintermann, B., and V. Valderrabano. 2003. Total ankle replacement. *Foot Ankle Clin.* 8:375–405.

Jaakkola, J. I., and R. A. Mann. 2004. A review of rheumatoid arthritis affecting the foot and ankle. *Foot Ankle Int.* 25:866–874.

Jarvinen, T. A., P. Kannus, N. Maffulli, and K. M. Khan. 2005. Achilles tendon disorders: Etiology and epidemiology. *Foot Ankle Clin.* 10:255–266.

Keiserman, L. S., V. J. Sammarco, and G. J. Sammarco. 2005. Surgical treatment of the hallux rigidus. *Foot Ankle Clin.* 10:75–96.

Krishna, Sayana M., and N. Maffulli. 2005. Insertional Achilles tendinopathy. *Foot Ankle Clin.* 10:309–320.

Marks, R. M. 2005. Arthrodesis of the first metatarsophalangeal joint. *Instr Course Lect.* 54:263–268.

McGuire, J. B. 2003. Arthritis and related diseases of the foot and ankle: Rehabilitation and biomechanical considerations. *Clin Podiatr Med Surg.* 20:469–485.

Melhus, A. 2005. Fluoroquinolones and tendon disorders. *Expert Opin Drug Saf.* 4:299–309.

Michelson, J. D. 2003. Ankle fractures resulting from rotational injuries. *J Am Acad Orthop Surg.* 11:403–412.

Miller, R. A., T. A. Decoster, and M. S. Mizel. 2005. What's new in foot and ankle surgery. *J Bone Joint Surg Am.* 87:909–917.

Mizel, M. S., P. J. Hecht, J. V. Marymont, and H. T. Temple. 2004. Evaluation and treatment of chronic ankle pain. *Instr Course Lect.* 53:311–321.

Mosier-LaClair, S., H. Pike, and G. Pomeroy. 2002. Syndesmosis injuries: Acute, chronic, new techniques for failed management. *Foot Ankle Clin.* 7:551–565.

Movin, T., A. Ryberg, D. J. McBride, and N. Maffulli. 2005. Acute rupture of the Achilles tendon. *Foot Ankle Clin.* 10:331–356.

Muir, D. C., A. Amendola, and C. L. Saltzman. 2002. Long-term outcome of ankle arthrodesis. *Foot Ankle Clin.* 7:703–708.

Mullen, J. E., and M. J. O'Malley. 2004. Sprains—Residual instability of subtalar, Lisfranc joints, and turf toe. *Clin Sports Med.* 23:97–121.

Norkus, S. A., and R. T. Floyd. 2001. The anatomy and mechanisms of syndesmotic ankle sprains. *J Athl Train.* 36:68–73.

O'Brien, M. 2005. The anatomy of the Achilles tendon. *Foot Ankle Clin.* 10:225–238.

Osborne, M. D., and T. D. Rizzo, Jr. 2003. Prevention and treatment of ankle sprain in athletes. *Sports Med.* 33:1145–1150.

Paavola, M., P. Kannus, T. A. Jarvinen, K. Khan, L. Jozsa, and M. Jarvinen. 2002. Achilles tendinopathy. *J Bone Joint Surg Am.* 84:2062–2076.

Pijnenburg, A. C., K. Bogaard, R. Krips, R. K. Marti, P. M. Bossuyt, and C. N. van Dijk. 2003. Operative and functional treatment of rupture of the lateral ligament of the ankle: A randomised, prospective trial. *J Bone Joint Surg Br.* 85:525–530.

Sammarco, V. J., and R. Nichols. 2005. Orthotic management for disorders of the hallux. *Foot Ankle Clin.* 10:191–209.

Specchiulli, F., and R. Mangialardi. 2004. The surgical treatment of

malleolar fractures: Long-term results. *Chir Organi Mov.* 89:313–
318.

Speed, C. A. 2004. Extracorporeal shock-wave therapy in the management of chronic soft-tissue conditions. *J Bone Joint Surg Br.* 86:165–
171.

Struijs, P., and G. Kerkhoffs. 2005. Ankle sprain. *Clin Evid.* 13:1366–
1376.

Thomas, R. H., and T. R. Daniels. 2003. Ankle arthritis. *J Bone Joint
Surg Am.* 85:923–936.

Thordarson, D. B. 2004. Fusion in posttraumatic foot and ankle reconstruction. *J Am Acad Orthop Surg.* 12:322–333.

Van Dijk, C. N. 2002. Management of the sprained ankle. *Br J Sports
Med.* 36:83–84.

Van Os, A. G., S. M. Bierma-Zeinstra, A. P. Verhagen, R. A. de Bie,
P. A. Luijsterburg, and B. W. Koes. 2005. Comparison of conventional treatment and supervised rehabilitation for treatment of acute
lateral ankle sprains: A systematic review of the literature. *J Orthop
Sports Phys Ther.* 35:95–105.

Williams, S. K., and M. Brage. 2004. Heel pain-plantar fasciitis and
Achilles enthesopathy. *Clin Sports Med.* 23:123–144.

Young, J. S., S. M. Kumta, and N. Maffulli. 2005. Achilles tendon rupture and tendinopathy: Management of complications. *Foot Ankle
Clin.* 10:371–382.

Zoch, C., V. Fialka-Moser, and M. Quittan. 2003. Rehabilitation of ligamentous ankle injuries: A review of recent studies. *Br J Sports Med.*
37:291–295.

Chapter 5. The Shoulder

Chambler, A. F., and A. J. Carr. 2003. The role of surgery in frozen
shoulder. *J Bone Joint Surg Br.* 85:789–795.

Cordasco, F. A., S. Steinmann, E. L. Flatow, and L. U. Bigliani. 1993.
Arthroscopic treatment of glenoid labral tears. *Am J Sports Med.*
21:425–430.

Dias, R., S. Cutts, and S. Massoud. 2005. Frozen shoulder. *BMJ.*
331:1453–1456.

Farrell, C. M., J. W. Sperling, and R. H. Cofield. 2005. Manipulation for
frozen shoulder: Long-term results. *J Shoulder Elbow Surg.* 14:480–
484.

Gartsman, G. M. 2001. All arthroscopic rotator cuff repairs. *Orthop Clin North Am.* 32:501–510.

Green, A. 1998. Current concepts of shoulder arthroplasty. *Instr Course Lect.* 47:127–133.

Green, A. 2003. Chronic massive rotator cuff tears: Evaluation and management. *J Am Acad Orthop Surg.* 11:321–331.

Grey, R. G. 1978. The natural history of "idiopathic" frozen shoulder. *J Bone Joint Surg Am.* 60:564.

Hovelius, L. 1982. Incidence of shoulder dislocation in Sweden. *Clin Orthop Relat Res.* 166:127–131.

Hovelius, L., B. G. Augustini, H. Fredin, O. Johansson, R. Norlin, and J. Thorling. 1996. Primary anterior dislocation of the shoulder in young patients: A ten-year prospective study. *J Bone Joint Surg Am.* 78:1677–1684.

Ide, J., S. Maeda, and K. Takagi. 2005. A comparison of arthroscopic and open rotator cuff repair. *Arthroscopy.* 21:1090–1098.

Itoi, E., Y. Hatakeyama, T. Kido, T. Sato, H. Minagawa, I. Wakabayashi, and M. Kobayashi M. 2003. A new method of immobilization after traumatic anterior dislocation of the shoulder: A preliminary study. *J Shoulder Elbow Surg.* 12:413–415.

Kannus, P., and A. Natri. 1997. Etiology and pathophysiology of tendon ruptures in sports. *Scand J Med Sci Sports.* 7:107–112.

Kim, S. H., and K. I. Ha. 2000. Arthroscopic treatment of symptomatic shoulders with minimally displaced greater tuberosity fracture. *Arthroscopy.* 16:695–700.

Lintner, S. A., and K. P. Speer. 1997. Traumatic anterior glenohumeral instability: The role of arthroscopy. *J Am Acad Orthop Surg.* 5:233–239.

Lo, I. K., J. Y. Bishop, A. Miniaci, and E. L. Flatow. 2004. Multi-directional instability: Surgical decision making. *Instr Course Lect.* 53:565–572.

Magee, T., D. Williams, and N. Mani. 2004. Shoulder MR arthrography: Which patient group benefits most. *AJR Am J Roentgenol.* 183:969–974.

Mantone, J. K., W. Z. Burkhead, Jr., and J. Noonan, Jr. 2000. Nonoperative treatment of rotator cuff tears. *Orthop Clin North Am.* 31:295–311.

Musgrave, D. S., and M. W. Rodosky. 2001. SLAP lesions: Current concepts. *Am J Orthop.* 30:29–38.

Ogilvie-Harris, D. J., D. J. Biggs, D. P. Fitsialos, and M. MacKay. 1995.

The resistant frozen shoulder: Manipulation versus arthroscopic release. *Clin Orthop Relat Res.* 319:238–248.

Pearl, M. L., A. A. Romeo, M. A. Wirth, K. Yamaguchi, G. P. Nicholson, and R. A. Creighton. 2005. Decision making in contemporary shoulder arthroplasty. *Instr Course Lect.* 54:69–85.

Pearsall, A. W., and K. P. Speer. 1998. Frozen shoulder syndrome: diagnostic and treatment strategies in the primary care setting. *Med Sci Sports Exerc.* 30:33–39.

Reeves, B. 1975. The natural history of the frozen shoulder syndrome. *Scand J Rheumatol.* 4:193–196.

Rowe, C. R. 1980. Acute and recurrent anterior dislocations of the shoulder. *Orthop Clin North Am.* 11:253–270.

Snyder, S. J. 1993. Evaluation and treatment of the rotator cuff. *Orthop Clin North Am.* 24:173–192.

Snyder, S. J., R. P. Karzel, W. Del Pizzo, R. D. Ferkel, and M. J. Friedman. 1990. SLAP lesions of the shoulder. *Arthroscopy.* 6:274–279.

Torchia, M. E., R. H. Cofield, and C. R. Settergren. 1997. Total shoulder arthroplasty with the Neer prosthesis: Long-term results. *J Shoulder Elbow Surg.* 6:495–505.

Toyoda, H., Y. Ito, H. Tomo, Y. Nakao, T. Koike, and K. Takaoka. 2005. Evaluation of rotator cuff tears with magnetic resonance arthrography. *Clin Orthop Relat Res.* 439:109–115.

Williams, G. R., Jr., C. A. Rockwood, Jr., L. U. Bigliani, J. P. Iannotti, and W. Stanwood. 2004. Rotator cuff tears: Why do we repair them? *J Bone Joint Surg Am.* 86:2764–2776.

Woodward, T. W., and T. M. Best. 2000. The painful shoulder: Part II. Acute and chronic disorders. *Am Fam Physician.* 61:3291–3300.

Youm, T., D. H. Murray, E. N. Kubiak, A. S. Rokito, and J. D. Zuckerman. 2005. Arthroscopic versus mini-open rotator cuff repair: A comparison of clinical outcomes and patient satisfaction. *J Shoulder Elbow Surg.* 14:455–459.

Chapter 6. The Elbow

Chen, F. S., A. S. Rokito, and F. W. Jobe. 2001. Medial elbow problems in the overhead-throwing athlete. *J Am Acad Orthop Surg.* 9:99–113.

Ciccotti, M. C., M. A. Schwartz, and M. G. Ciccotti. 2004. Diagnosis and treatment of medial epicondylitis of the elbow. *Clin Sports Med.* 23:693–705.

Gruchow, H. W., and D. Pelletier. 1979. An epidemiologic study of tennis elbow: Incidence, recurrence, and effectiveness of prevention strategies. *Am J Sports Med.* 7:234–238.

Hargreaves, D., and R. Emery. 1999. Total elbow replacement in the treatment of rheumatoid disease. *Clin Orthop Relat Res.* 366:61–71.

Jobe, F. W., and M. G. Ciccotti. 1994. Lateral and medial epicondylitis of the elbow. *J Am Acad Orthop Surg.* 2:1–8.

Leach, R. E., and J. K. Miller. 1987. Lateral and medial epicondylitis of the elbow. *Clin Sports Med.* 6:259–272.

McLaughlin, R. E., II, F. H. Savoie, III, L. D. Field, and J. R. Ramsey. 2006. Arthroscopic treatment of the arthritic elbow due to primary radiocapitellar arthritis. *Arthroscopy.* 22:63–69.

Nirschl, R. P., and E. S. Ashman. 2004. Tennis elbow tendinosis (epicondylitis). *Instr Course Lect.* 53:587–598.

Nirschl, R. P., and F. A. Pettrone. 1979. Tennis elbow: The surgical treatment of lateral epicondylitis. *J Bone Joint Surg Am.* 61:832–839.

O'Driscoll, S. W. 1993. Elbow arthritis: Treatment options. *J Am Acad Orthop Surg.* 1:106–116.

O'Driscoll, S. W., J. B. Jupiter, G. J. King, R. N. Hotchkiss, and B. F. Morrey. 2001. The unstable elbow. *Instr Course Lect.* 50:89–102.

Rompe J. D., C. Theis, and N. Maffulli. 2005. Shock wave treatment for tennis elbow. *Orthopade.* 34:567–570.

Salzman, K. L., W. A. Lillegard, and J. D. Butcher. 1997. Upper extremity bursitis. *Am Fam Physician.* 56:1797–1806.

Sellards, R., and C. Kuebrich. 2005. The elbow: Diagnosis and treatment of common injuries. *Prim Care.* 32:1–16.

Smith, D. L., J. H. McAfee, L. M. Lucas, K. L. Kumar, and D. M. Romney. 1989. Treatment of nonseptic olecranon bursitis: A controlled, blinded prospective trial. *Arch Intern Med.* 11:2527–2530.

Steinmann, S. P., G. J. King, F. H. Savoie, III. 2005. American Academy of Orthopaedic Surgeons: Arthroscopic treatment of the arthritic elbow. *J Bone Joint Surg Am.* 87:2114–2121.

Stewart, N. J., J. B. Manzanares, and B. F. Morrey. 1997. Surgical treatment of aseptic olecranon bursitis. *J Shoulder Elbow Surg.* 6:49–54.

Thompson, G. R., B. M. Manshady, and J. J. Weiss. 1978. Septic bursitis. *JAMA.* 240:2280–2281.

Williams, R. J., III, E. R. Urquhart, and D. W. Altchek. 2004. Medial collateral ligament tears in the throwing athlete. *Instr Course Lect.* 53:579–586.

Wilson, J. J., and T. M. Best. 2005. Common overuse tendon problems: A review and recommendations for treatment. *Am Fam Physician.* 72:811–818.

Chapter 7. The Hand and Wrist

Abboud, J. A., P. K. Beredjiklian, and D. J. Bozentka. 2003. Metacarpophalangeal joint arthroplasty in rheumatoid arthritis. *J Am Acad Orthop Surg.* 11:184–191.

Adams, B. D. 2004. Surgical management of the arthritic wrist. *Instr Course Lect.* 53:41–45.

Akhtar, S., M. J. Bradley, D. N. Quinton, and F. D. Burke. 2005. Management and referral for trigger finger/thumb. *BMJ.* 331:30–33.

Ashworth, N. 2004. Carpal tunnel syndrome. *Clin Evid.* 12:1558–1577.

Bendre, A. A., B. J. Hartigan, and D. M. Kalainov. 2005. Mallet finger. *J Am Acad Orthop Surg.* 13:336–344.

Burke, F. D., J. Ellis, H. McKenna, and M. J. Bradley. 2003. Primary care management of carpal tunnel syndrome. *Postgrad Med J.* 79:433–437.

Chan, D. Y. 2002. Management of simple finger injuries: The splinting regime. *Hand Surg.* 7:223–230.

Cooney, W. P., III. 2003. Scaphoid fractures: current treatments and techniques. *Instr Course Lect.* 52:197–208.

Hausman, M. 2004. Conservative surgical treatment of wrist arthritis. *Instr Course Lect.* 53:23–30.

Hodge, D. K., and M. R. Safran. 2002. Sideline management of common dislocations. *Curr Sports Med Rep.* 1:149–155.

Ilan, D. I., and M. E. Rettig. 2003. Rheumatoid arthritis of the wrist. *Bull Hosp Jt Dis.* 61:179–185.

Lee, S. G, and J. B. Jupiter. 2000. Phalangeal and metacarpal fractures of the hand. *Hand Clin.* 16:323–332.

MacDermid, J. C., and J. Wessel. 2004. Clinical diagnosis of carpal tunnel syndrome: A systematic review. *J Hand Ther.* 17:309–319.

McAuliffe, J. A., and R. S. Carneiro. 1998. Inflammatory and traumatic tendinopathies about the ulnar wrist. *Hand Clin.* 14:317–326.

Michlovitz, S. L. 2004. Conservative interventions for carpal tunnel syndrome. *J Orthop Sports Phys Ther.* 34:589–600.

Nahra, M. E., and J. S. Bucchieri. 2004. Ganglion cysts and other tumor related conditions of the hand and wrist. *Hand Clin.* 20:249–260.

Norregaard, O., J. Jakobsen, and K. K. Nielsen. 1987. Hyperextension injuries of the PIP finger joint: Comparison of early motion and immobilization. *Acta Orthop Scand.* 58:239–240.

Phillips, T. G., A. M. Reibach, and W. P. Slomiany. 2004. Diagnosis and management of scaphoid fractures. *Am Fam Physician.* 70:879–884.

Rettig, A. C. 2001. Wrist and hand overuse syndromes. *Clin Sports Med.* 20:591–611.

Ruch, D. S., A. J. Weiland, S. W. Wolfe, W. B. Geissler, M. S. Cohen, and J. B. Jupiter. 2004. Current concepts in the treatment of distal radial fractures. *Instr Course Lect.* 53:389–401.

Saldana, M. J. 2001. Trigger digits: Diagnosis and treatment. *J Am Acad Orthop Surg.* 9:246–252.

Shin, A. Y., M. A. Deitch, K. Sachar, and M. I. Boyer. 2005. Ulnar-sided wrist pain: Diagnosis and treatment. *Instr Course Lect.* 54:115–128.

Tallia, A. F., and D. A. Cardone. 2003. Diagnostic and therapeutic injection of the wrist and hand region. *Am Fam Physician.* 67:745–750.

Thoma, A., K. Veltri, T. Haines, and E. Duku. 2004. A systematic review of reviews comparing the effectiveness of endoscopic and open carpal tunnel decompression. *Plast Reconstr Surg.* 113:1184–1191.

Viera, A. J. 2003. Management of carpal tunnel syndrome. *Am Fam Physician.* 68:265–272.

Weiss, A. P. 2004. Osteoarthritis of the wrist. *Instr Course Lect.* 53:31–40.

Chapter 8. Common Medications and How They Work

Clegg, D. O., D. J. Reda, C. L. Harris, M. A. Klein, J. R. O'Dell, M. M. Hooper, J. D. Bradley, et al. 2006. Glucosamine, chondroitin sulfate, and the two in combination for painful knee osteoarthritis. *N Engl J Med.* 354:795–808.

Egbunike, I. G., and B. J. Chaffee. 1990. Antidepressants in the management of chronic pain syndromes. *Pharmacotherapy.* 10:262–270.

Fitzgerald, G. A. 2004. Coxibs and cardiovascular disease. *N Engl J Med.* 351:1709–1711.

Gass, M., and B. Dawson-Hughes. 2006. Preventing osteoporosis-related fractures: An overview. *Am J Med.* 119:3–11.

Genovese, M. C. 2005. Biologic therapies in clinical development for the treatment of rheumatoid arthritis. *J Clin Rheumatol.* 3 (suppl): S45–54.

Greenspan, S. L., T. J. Beck, N. M. Resnick, R. Bhattacharya, and R. A.

Parker. 2005. Effect of hormone replacement, alendronate, or combination therapy on hip structural geometry: A 3-year, double-blind, placebo-controlled clinical trial. *J Bone Miner Res.* 20:1525–1532.

Hanesch, U., M. Pawlak, and J. J. McDougall. 2003. Gabapentin reduces the mechanosensitivity of fine afferent nerve fibres in normal and inflamed rat knee joints. *Pain.* 104:363–366.

Knowles, S. R., E. J. Phillips, G. Wong, and N. H. Shear. 2004. Serious dermatologic reaction associated with valdecoxib: Report of two cases. *J Am Acad Dermatol.* 51:1028–1029.

Konttinen, Y. T., S. Seitsalo, M. Lehto, and S. Santavirta. 2005. Current management: Management of rheumatic diseases in the era of biological anti-rheumatic drugs. *Acta Orthop.* 76:614–619.

Mahowald, M. L., J. A. Singh, and P. Majeski. 2005. Opioid use by patients in an orthopedics spine clinic. *Arthritis Rheum.* 52:312–321.

Moskowitz, R. W., M. A. Kelly, D. G. Lewallen, and C. T. Vangsness, Jr. 2004. Nonsurgical approaches to pain management for osteoarthritis of the knee. *Am J Orthop.* 33:10–14.

Nicholson B. 2003. Responsible prescribing of opioids for the management of chronic pain. *Drugs.* 63:17–32.

NIII Consensus Development Panel on Osteoporosis Prevention, Diagnosis, and Therapy. 2001. Osteoporosis prevention, diagnosis, and therapy. *JAMA.* 285:785–795.

Rozental, T. D., and T. P. Sculco. 2000. Intra-articular corticosteroids: An updated overview. *Am J Orthop.* 29:18–23.

Schieffer, B. M., Q. Pham, J. Labus, A. Baria, W. Van Vort, P. Davis, F. Davis, and B. D. Naliboff. 2005. Pain medication beliefs and medication misuse in chronic pain. *J Pain.* 6:620–629.

Schnitzer, T. J. 1998. Non-NSAID pharmacologic treatment options for the management of chronic pain. *Am J Med.* 105:45S–52S.

Todd, C. 2002. Meeting the therapeutic challenge of the patient with osteoarthritis. *J Am Pharm Assoc* (Wash). 42:74–82.

Vane, J. R., and R. M. Botting. 2003. The mechanism of action of aspirin. *Thromb Res.* 110:255–258.

Chapter 9. When to Consider a Joint Injection

Atamaz, F., Y. Kirazli, and Y. Akkoc. 2006. A comparison of two different intra-articular hyaluronan drugs and physical therapy in the management of knee osteoarthritis. *Rheumatol Int.* 26:873–878.

Bang, M. S., and S. H. Lim. 2006. Paraplegia caused by spinal infection after acupuncture. *Spinal Cord.* 44:258–259.

Barnes, P. M., E. Powell-Griner, K. McFann, and R. L. Nahin. 2004. Complementary and alternative medicine use among adults: United States, 2002. *Adv Data.* 343:1–19.

Berman, B. M., L. Lao, P. Langenberg, W. L. Lee, A. M. Gilpin, and M. C. Hochberg. 2004. Effectiveness of acupuncture as adjunctive therapy in osteoarthritis of the knee: A randomized, controlled trial. *Ann Intern Med.* 141:901–910.

Campbell, D. G., K. R. Angel, P. J. Dobson, P. L. Lewis, and S. Tandon. 2004. Experiences of viscosupplementation for knee osteoarthritis. *Aust Fam Physician.* 33:863–864.

Eisenberg, D. M., R. C. Kessler, C. Foster, F. E. Norlock, D. R. Calkins, and T. L. Delbanco. 1993. Unconventional medicine in the United States: Prevalence, costs, and patterns of use. *N Engl J Med.* 328:246–252.

Goldberg, V. M., and R. D. Coutts. 2004. Pseudoseptic reactions to hylan viscosupplementation: Diagnosis and treatment. *Clin Orthop Relat Res.* 419:130–137.

Gomis, A., M. Pawlak, E. A. Balazs, R. F. Schmidt, and C. Belmonte. 2004. Effects of different molecular weight elastoviscous hyaluronan solutions on articular nociceptive afferents. *Arthritis Rheum.* 50:314–326.

Han, J. S. 2004. Acupuncture and endorphins. *Neurosci Lett.* 361:258–261.

Karatay, S., A. Kiziltunc, K. Yildirim, R. C. Karanfil, and K. Senel. 2004. Effects of different hyaluronic acid products on synovial fluid levels of intercellular adhesion molecule-1 and vascular cell adhesion molecule-1 in knee osteoarthritis. *Ann Clin Lab Sci.* 34:330–335.

Lo, G. H., M. LaValley, T. McAlindon, and D. T. Felson. 2003. Intra-articular hyaluronic acid in treatment of knee osteoarthritis: a meta-analysis. *JAMA.* 290:3115–3121.

Migliore, A., S. Tormenta, L. S. Martin, F. Iannessi, U. Massafra, E. Carloni, D. Monno, A. Alimonti, and M. Granata. 2006. The symptomatic effects of intra-articular administration of hylan G-F 20 on osteoarthritis of the hip: Clinical data of 6 months follow-up. *Clin Rheumatol.* 25(3):389–93

Nahleh, Z., and I. A. Tabbara. 2003. Complementary and alternative medicine in breast cancer patients. *Palliat Support Care.* 1:267–273.

Patrick, B. S. 2005. Acupuncture complication—a case report. *J Miss State Med Assoc.* 46:195–197.

Chapter 10. Alternative Therapies

Sherman, K. J., D. C. Cherkin, D. M. Eisenberg, J. Erro, A. Hrbek, and R. A. Deyo. 2005. The practice of acupuncture: Who are the providers and what do they do. *Ann Fam Med.* 3:151–158.

Tindle, H. A., R. B. Davis, R. S. Phillips, and D. M. Eisenberg. 2005. Trends in use of complementary and alternative medicine by U.S. adults: 1997–2002. *Altern Ther Health Med.* 11:42–49.

Wetzel, M. S., D. M. Eisenberg, and T. J. Kaptchuk. 1998. Courses involving complementary and alternative medicine at U.S. medical schools. *JAMA.* 280:784–787.

Windhorst, C. E. 1998. Alternative medicine's potent attraction for boomers and seniors. *Health Strateg.* 10:7–8.

Witt, C., B. Brinkhaus, S. Jena, K. Linde, A. Streng, S. Wagenpfeil, J. Hummelsberger, H. U. Walther, D. Melchart, and S. N. Willich. 2005. Acupuncture in patients with osteoarthritis of the knee: A randomised trial. *Lancet.* 366:136–143.

Epilogue

Allroggen, A., A. Frese, A. Rahmann, M. Gaubitz, I. W. Husstedt, and S. Evers. 2005. HIV associated arthritis: Case report and review of the literature. *Eur J Med Res.* 10:305–308.

Dogne, J. M., J. Hanson, C. Supuran, and D. Pratico. 2006. Coxibs and cardiovascular side-effects: From light to shadow. *Curr Pharm Des.* 12:971–975.

Farahani, P., M. Levine, K. Gaebel, E. C. Wang, and N. Khalidi. 2006. Community-based evaluation of etanercept in patients with rheumatoid arthritis. *J Rheumatol.* 33:665–670.

Goss, R. J. 1969. *Principles of regeneration.* New York: Academic Press.

Haseltine, W. A. 2004. An interview with William A. Haseltine. *Rejuvenation Res.* 7:229–231.

Holmberg, S., A. Thelin, and N. Thelin. 2005. Knee osteoarthritis and body mass index: A population-based case-control study. *Scand J Rheumatol.* 34:59–64.

Hosaka, K., J. Ryu, S. Saitoh, T. Ishii, K. Kuroda, and K. Shimizu.

2005. The combined effects of anti-TNFalpha antibody and IL-1 receptor antagonist in human rheumatoid arthritis synovial membrane. *Cytokine*. 32:263–269.

Knowles, S. R., E. J. Phillips, G. Wong, and N. H. Shear. 2004. Serious dermatologic reaction associated with valdecoxib: Report of two cases. *J Am Acad Dermatol*. 51:1028–1029.

Murphy, G., and M. H. Lee. 2005. What are the roles of metallo-proteinases in cartilage and bone damage? *Ann Rheum Dis*. 64:44–47.

Roos, E. M. 2005. Joint injury causes knee osteoarthritis in young adults. *Curr Opin Rheumatol*. 17:195–200.

Yelin, E., C. Henke, and W. Epstein. 1987. The work dynamics of the person with rheumatoid arthritis. *Arthritis Rheum*. 30:507–512.

INDEX

Page numbers in *italics* indicate illustrations